PRAISE FOR LEIGH ELDER

An excellent book to inspire, motivate and help readers to improve their long-term health.
—*Arch Jelley, legendary athletics coach*

Leigh has grit, talks commonsense and has a powerful group of medical mentors backing his philosophies.
—*Robyn Langwell, NZ Herald*

Leigh is one of NZ's most successful – and most unlikely – weight loss gurus.
—*Donna Fleming, NZ Women's Weekly*

PRAISE FOR LEIGH'S EAT FOR KEEPS PROGRAMME

The Eat For Keeps Experience ... has great content and congrats to all involved.
—*Professor Jennie-Brand Miller, best-selling author of the New Glucose Revolution book series*

I have been an adviser to EFK for a number of years and this is a programme I would support the full development of.
—*Professor Cliff-Tasman Jones, clinical nutrition specialist and founder of the NZ Nutrition Foundation*

We regularly use EFK in our practice and its principles are a

powerful force in helping improve or reverse many type 2 diabetic conditions and obesity.
—*Dr Trish Zingel, Tauranga*

We both lend and sell the EFK books in our practice, I personally agree with these concepts and have seen many people do really well using them.
—*Dr Kevin Giles, Mt Maunganui, recently retired*

In August 2013, I was a 91.5 kg insulin-dependent, asthmatic. I was on four injections of almost 100 units of insulin a day and blood pressure, cholesterol, reflux, thyroid and asthma medication. I met Leigh Elder, started following both the Eat For Keeps concepts and my new GP's guidelines. The only medication I take now is thyroxin and enjoy a healthy weight and life free from diabetes.
—*Penny Pelan, Queensland*

One of my greatest challenges has been to overcome a serious weight problem which has led to diabetes. I consulted a number of health professionals and tried a number of diets but could not make any headway. In 2009 I had a consultation with EFK founder, Leigh Elder. I now have a really clear view on how and why I put on weight and have the skills and know-how to manage my weight, even when travelling around the world. I have lost about 15 kg and my diabetes is now under control.
—*Tony Christiansen, Mt Maunganui), double amputee, world-class motivational speaker*

DON'T ACT YOUR AGE

Living Younger Can Be Age-defying

LEIGH ELDER

Copyright © 2025 Leigh Elder

Leigh Elder asserts his moral right to be identified as the author of this work.

All rights reserved. No part of this publication may be reproduced or transmitted in any form or by any means, electronic or mechanical, including photocopying, recording or information storage and retrieval systems, without permission in writing from the copyright holder.

Published by Kik Books

Author contact: https://leighelder.substack.com or leighelderwriter@gmail.com

A catalogue record for this book is available from the National Library of New Zealand.

ISBN 978-0-473-75648-2 (paperback)
ISBN 978-0-473-75649-9 (EPUB)

CONTENTS

Introduction   xiii

Part One
LIFESTYLE MATTERS

1. **THE MIND GAME**   3
   - Key Points   3
   - Mind over matter   4
   - Getting clarity   5
   - Biological age   6
   - Healthspan   7
   - My personal challenge   8
   - Slowing the slide   9

2. **WHERE DO YOU STAND?**   10
   - Key Points   10
   - Accepting finality   11
   - Take a snapshot   11
   - Imagining the changes   13
   - Stick to your guns   14
   - Your incredible body   15
   - Gratitude   16
   - Irene's story   16

3. **CELEBRATE MOVEMENT**   21
   - Key Points   21
   - The gift of movement   22
   - Proprioception   23
   - Made for movement   24
   - Fitness and health   25
   - Make any movement an opportunity   26
   - Celebrating all movement   27
   - Down with sitting   27

Regular movement and exercise	27
Pat's story	28

4. IN SEARCH OF HAPPINESS — 33
Key Points	33
Choosing how we live	34
The importance of gaining clarity	36
A happiness index	37
The four pillars	39
FOMO vs JOMO	40

5. HAVING THE RIGHT ATTITUDE — 43
Key Points	43
A DIY approach to healthcare	44
Are you ready?	45
Reviewing	46
Being prepared	47
June's story	48
Positivity	54
Focus on what you can control	55
Glass half full	56
Socially engaged	56
Purpose and challenge	57

6. SPORT AND OTHER LEISURE ACTIVITIES — 59
Key Points	59
Walking wonders	60
Walking quality versus quantity	63
Developing a walking plan	64
Other sports and pastimes	65
Vic's story	67

7. BUILDING RESILIENCE — 74
Key Points	74
Bouncing back	75
Ten traits of resilient people	76
Sherilyn's story	85

Part Two
PHYSICAL AND BIOLOGICAL MATTERS

1. PHYSICAL FUNCTIONALITY	**99**
Key Points	99
Physical Functionality (PF) and BAFFS	101
Life gets in the way	102
Fight back	103
Reality check	104
2. THE PHYSICAL FOUNDATION BLOCKS	**107**
Key Points	107
Gradual loss	108
The good news	109
Get all the BAFFS in one go	111
3. MANAGING YOUR PHYSICAL HEALTH	**112**
Key Points	112
Managing your health	114
General practitioner	115
Physiotherapist	119
DIY helps	120
Safety	121
Other health professionals	121
Summary: choosing a health professional	122
Health insurance	123
Medications	124
DIY mentality	127
Your physical health	127
Arch Jelley's story	131
Summing up Arch	148
4. MANAGING YOUR MENTAL HEALTH	**152**
Key Points	152
Facing challenges, embracing reality	153
Being grateful	155
Digital issues	156
Depression	157
Margaret Borland's story	158

5. HORMONES, METABOLIC SYNDROME AND
   DIETARY SUPPLEMENTS   170
   Key Points   170
   Hormones   171
   Metabolic Syndrome   174
   Dietary supplements   175
   Vitamin D   178
   Electrolytes   178
   Other vitamins   179
   Blood test   180

6. DEALING WITH INJURIES AND
   OTHER ACHES AND PAINS   181
   Key Points   181
   Types of injuries   182
   Nordic walking   186
   Tennis balls   187
   Understanding anatomy   188
   Some common ailments   189

7. LOWERING YOUR BIOLOGICAL AGE   196
   Key Points   196
   Forming new habits   197
   Biological vs chronological age   198
   Epigenetics   199
   Lowering your own biological age   201
   Super agers and not so super   202
   Taking the first step   204
   Reversing damage   206

Part Three
THE DON'T ACT YOUR AGE CHALLENGE
A Life-changing Challenge!

1. IMPROVING PHYSICAL FUNCTIONALITY (PF)   211
   Understanding and testing Your BAFFS   211
   Measuring your own BAFFS capabilities   213

Working out a BAFFS improvement plan for you	219
Summary	233
2. NUTRITION	235
Welcome to 'The EFK Method'	237
The EFK Way	245
Finally	248
3. BREAKING UP LONG PERIODS OF SITTING	249
4. DRINK FRESH WATER REGULARLY	254
5. BUILDING RESILIENCE	256
Ten traits of resilient people	257
WHAT TO DO NOW?	259
IN CONCLUSION	262
About the Author	265
Acknowledgments	267

To live is the rarest thing in the world.
Most people exist, that is all.
— Oscar Wilde

INTRODUCTION

Growing old is for so many a scary journey into the unknown. I understand this from my previous experience in owning a rest home and seeing the bewildered looks as new residents crossed our worthy threshold for the first time.

Many of these people were old before their time and suffering from one chronic illness or another as early as their late sixties and early seventies. They hated leaving the comfort of their own homes and familiar surroundings and were forced into it by their now despised lack of ability to live independently.

Those five poignant years have stayed with me. So often, if you didn't laugh, you'd cry. It was often heartbreaking seeing former high-functioning adults reduced to shadows of their former selves. Despite our fabulous staff's best efforts to provide great care, it was still a sad way for our residents to see out their days.

It was also sad to think that many of these people, if they had had the know-how and had made a few key lifestyle changes, could have easily got a decade or more of good health.

What a great reason for me to write a book which will help its readers to do exactly this, by showing them how to wind back their biological clocks.

In New Zealand, with an average life expectancy of eighty-two, the average time someone suffers a chronic illness is in their mid-sixties.

There is a lot at stake here. I feel I have to get this right. I'm reasonably well qualified to do this. I have a background in physical education teaching, life and business coaching, and have helped thousands of people with weight and diabetes issues. I have been a co-author of two popular *Eat For Keeps* books (manuals for people with weight and diabetes issues) and have contributed many newspaper columns.

SOME MOTIVATIONS

Apart from owning the rest home, there are other experiences that I have had in recent years which have motivated me to write this book.

Body Worlds

Gunther von Hagens' exhibition was one of these.

The skin was stripped away from cadavers to show what's underneath, and the bodies were displayed in many different, sometimes very athletic, poses. There were also cross sections of brains and all of our other organs, either in situ or suspended on their own.

I found the exhibition absolutely jaw dropping, and it made me instantly aware of this gift of life, these trillions of cells which include bones, muscles, tendons, hormones, nerves, and more. Most of us are given the near-perfect model, which allows us to breathe, move, smell, think, see, touch and feel.

Do you ever stop to think and be grateful to have been given this gift of life? I for one would have to admit that, more often than not, I don't.

Death denial

Another lightbulb moment was an enlightening conversation I had with my daughter-in-law Susan. She told me that most people go through their lives in a state of death denial.

They fail to acknowledge their inevitable demise and instead exist in a state where they feel immortal. This mental habit often results in them missing some of the key, subtle little changes that are happening in their bodies.

Death denial is definitely real, and I cover this subject in some detail.

Simple changes

Another defining experience happened during the years I was coaching people around weight and diabetes problems. What fascinated me was how quickly key medical markers improved when clients made a few simple lifestyle changes.

I recall many type 2 diabetics being able to stop injecting insulin and even reversing their condition after a few weeks of reducing their intake of simple and starchy carbohydrates.

This meant that some of the cellular damage to millions of cells in their circulatory system, liver, pancreas and other organs had been reversed. (Your biological age is actually assessed by the amount of damage done to your cells.)

This means that by making a few permanent lifestyle changes you can become biologically younger. How exciting is that?

The final chapter of my book is called The Don't Act Your Age

Challenge. It is a step-by-step guide to help you to increase your number of years of good health.

I write this book in the hope that I can help as many people as possible to become more aware of this gift of life. Also to help you realise that it is a once-only opportunity and that you can quite easily find ways to gain more years of good health.

WHAT *DON'T ACT YOUR AGE* IS ALL ABOUT

I believe that I have benefited immensely from taking a personal negative health situation a few years ago and turning it into a positive lifetime challenge.

I hated the idea of growing old and have turned this negative thought to my own advantage. In doing this I had to first delve into my own experiences and research all the available science I could find to help me to live younger.

Having twenty years' experience helping thousands of people with their weight and diabetes issues gave me a good head start. The Eat For Keeps programme had a high success rate of about 50 per cent and also meant I rubbed shoulders and learned a great deal from GPs, medical specialists and other health professionals.

This book is all about what I have learned, and it includes the superb and eye-opening contributions from a number of vibrant, optimistic and inspirational super-agers. They seem to have a glint in their eye, and they certainly do not act their age.

The ultimate formula for having the best chance of a lengthy, happy, fulfilling and healthy life is compelling and simple.

You can live longer by 'living younger'.

This book is full of simple, practical exercises and action steps. It also contains a number of brief life stories of people in their nineties and beyond. They are almost like case studies as these super-agers exhibit common characteristics which have helped them to live long and healthy lives.

I have found these people to be very inspiring and loved the notion that they all thought that I was quite a young fellow.

You can obviously read this book from cover to cover. If you want to be more selective, each chapter begins with a summary of some key points to help you decide whether the chapter contains topics of interest to you.

Part One
LIFESTYLE MATTERS

1
THE MIND GAME

KEY POINTS

- 'Mind over matter' is the situation where someone can get control of most physical conditions, situations or problems by using the mind.
- We subconsciously develop strategies to fend off the awareness of inevitable death and escape into the feeling that we are immortal.
- The key to getting your mind around how to get the best out of the rest of your life is to be absolutely clear how the rest of your life could look, and to make a plan of attack.
- Although your chronological age reflects certain expectations of your physical and mental health, your biological age can confound these expectations.
- Mental capability involves such basic things as the ability to read, write, understand basic concepts, have

functioning long and short-term memory, and do basic day-to-day activities like cooking, shopping and household chores.
- If you have higher levels of ability across this whole range than your chronological age expectation, your biological age will be correspondingly lower. If you have lower levels of ability, your biological age will be higher.
- 'Healthspan' is the total number of years you spend in good health, free from any chronic disease and disabilities associated with ageing.
- From age thirty your body starts to incrementally deteriorate. If you are prepared to make small positive changes to your lifestyle, you will slow down this slide.
- Are a few more years of good health, or perhaps even a decade or two, of this once-only chance you get on this planet worthwhile?

MIND OVER MATTER

'Getting your mind round it' and 'mind over matter' are common sayings. I believe that the mind lies at the heart of all things in your life and rightly takes pride of place as my first chapter.

'Mind over matter' is the situation where someone can get control of most physical conditions, situations or problems by using the mind.

Although genetics and fate play their part, your brain will otherwise totally dominate the entire landscape of your life. It will determine your ultimate successes or failures, happiness or sadness.

The Denial of Death is the title of Ernest Becker's best-known book, which won the Pulitzer Prize in 1974. He believes that we subconsciously develop strategies to fend off awareness of our inevitable death and escape into the feeling that we're immortal.

This is a classic case of our minds being programmed over time to conveniently believe this. And I believe Becker has identified an incredibly common state of mind. This inability to face the reality of your inevitable demise provides a major stumbling block and ultimately often prevents you taking responsibility for your physical health.

This 'she'll be right' mentality sometimes blocks the necessity for you to take positive action to prevent impending health issues.

GETTING CLARITY

The key to getting your mind around how to get the best out of the rest of your life is to get absolute clarity on how the rest of your life could look, and to make a plan of attack.

In 2021 Kate and I moved into a new retirement village in Devonport. I was seventy-seven at the time and had to get my mind around the idea that this was 99 per cent likely to be our final home. After many shifts to different towns and cities over my lifetime, this finality took a while to sink in.

Simultaneously, and in lieu of this finality, I started to think about my own mortality for the first time. I had three years to go until reaching the average life expectancy age of eighty for New Zealand men. Wow, I thought, if I'm average, I have already lived over 95 per cent of my life. Well, okay, I am pretty fit and healthy, so if I were to get to ninety, this reduces to 86 per cent. I thought that even reaching the age of 100 only leaves me with 23 per cent of my life left.

My eldest son is fifty-eight. If he were to live until he is ninety, he will already have lived 65 per cent of his life. Quite scarily, he's already lived 72 per cent to reach the average life expectancy.

This numerical reality certainly puts your life into perspective and makes a dent in any death-denial tendencies you may have.

BIOLOGICAL AGE

The next step in this rewiring process is to understand the term biological age.

Although your chronological age informs certain expectations of your physical and mental health, your biological age can confound these expectations. *Estimations of biological age find that these can vary from between being many years younger to being years older than your chronological age.*

Biological age indicates how rapidly or slowly a person is ageing. Some of the factors involved in assessing biological age include:

- **Physical state** – This includes key factors like strength, flexibility, cardiovascular fitness, balance, agility, walking speed (time taken to walk a specified distance) and weight.
- **Mental capability** – Ability to read, write, understand basic concepts, have functioning long and short-term memory and be able to perform basic day-to-day activities like cooking, shopping and household chores; these are some of the basics.
- **Biological health** – This is the overall health of the cells of your body including in the circulatory system, nervous system, organs and all of the other structures.

If you have higher levels of function across this whole range than your chronological age expectation, your cellular health will reflect this, and your biological age will be correspondingly lower. If you have poorer levels of cellular health, your biological age will be higher.

The advantages of having a biological age lower than your chronological age are obvious.

This chapter is about getting your mind around how the rest of your life could play out to your best advantage. The rest of this book is about helping you to have the best opportunity of having a biological age lower than your chronological age. Believe me, this is a goal worth pursuing.

HEALTHSPAN

This leads us on to one final and highly related concept called healthspan. *This is the total number of years you spend in good health, free from any chronic disease and disabilities associated with ageing.*

If you can have a biological age which is significantly lower than your chronological age, your healthspan years will correspondingly increase.

In the years when my age was pushing up towards seventy, I can distinctly remember thinking to myself that I was not going to have a bar of all this ageing business.

We were living in Mount Maunganui, which is both a scenic and lively North Island coastal resort town. It is a brilliant place to not act your age – and we didn't. We had a very active group of friends and regular interests included golf, tennis, kayaking, biking, swimming and walking."

At the same time during this period, some health scares came my way, and I needed a bowel resection to get rid of a potentially cancerous lesion. I also had other minor ops including for skin lesions, knee arthroscopy, and an inguinal hernia. More latterly, a huge scare for me was a melanoma, which was removed from my head.

I have been so lucky to date to have emerged from all these with a fairly clean slate, although who knows what is around the corner? All of this will be familiar territory for any readers who are aged north of sixty.

I think that my bowel op was a defining moment for me. I began to realise that I was not immortal after all, and this sentiment was reinforced by the loss of three of our close friends in their early seventies to either cancer or heart disease. These untimely deaths hit our tight-knit group of friends hard.

MY PERSONAL CHALLENGE

The result of this defining moment was to make a conscious decision to add another challenge to the list of the many sports and pastimes I have participated in over my lifetime.

I challenged myself to become the best I could reasonably be for the rest of my life. 'Reasonably' being the objective word. I had always been a social drinker, and this was not about to change.

And so, I had got my mind around it. *I was no longer in death denial. Instead, I had a specific and measurable challenge ahead, which would always acknowledge my eventual demise.*

The challenge was to be able to wring as many years of good health out of myself as possible. My key mantra became, 'I am going to live my life like someone who is twenty years younger than me, and with a biological age to match.'

Parts of the rest of this book are about how I have gone about this, what I have learned and where I have got up to. I hope you too can reap some benefits from these many and varied experiences.

SLOWING THE SLIDE

From age thirty your body starts to incrementally deteriorate. If you are prepared to make small positive changes to your lifestyle, you will slow this downward slide.

This means that you are highly likely to lower your biological age and increase the number of your healthspan years. Are a few more years of good health, or perhaps even a decade or two, worthwhile?

Some of the inspiring personal stories you will read will certainly give you a good idea of what's possible.

It's all just a matter of getting your mind around it!

2
WHERE DO YOU STAND?

KEY POINTS

- Accepting that your life does have a final deadline and consigning 'death denial' to the scrap heap is a crucial step forward in getting the best out of the rest of your life. This will allow you to appreciate the value of increasing your healthspan years.
- Once you recognise and accept that 'shit happens', and that you just have to deal with it, it can make life easier. Also recognise that some things are out of your control and therefore not worth worrying about.
- If you are keen to start making a few changes, take a realistic attitude and recognise and accept that you probably will suffer some setbacks along the way.
- Also be wary of the old trap of starting off with massive enthusiasm and gradually slackening off as all of life's

other challenges get in the way. Be staunch and stick to your guns.
- Another important idea is to be grateful for this gift of life. How could you possibly just take it for granted or, worse still, neglect it?
- Your challenge can take any shape you like and will of course reflect your various strengths and weaknesses.

Having just read that first chapter, you will no doubt be having some thoughts on how to get the best out of the rest of your life.

ACCEPTING FINALITY

Accepting that your life does have a final deadline, and consigning 'death denial' to the scrap heap, is a crucial step forward.

This will allow you to appreciate the value of increasing your healthspan years. It will also give you the opportunity to slow down and sometimes reverse the incremental decline you will naturally experience after age thirty.

As a result, you will lower your biological age and 'add life to your years and very likely years to your life'. Even though this is a hackneyed phrase, it is oh so true.

I hope you are intrigued and a bit excited about how you could positively reinvent yourself. The rest of the chapter is about helping you to make a start and figure out how you are going to go about it.

TAKE A SNAPSHOT

A great place to start and a compelling reality check is to take a snapshot of where you are up to with your life. Let's look at how you can do this in a physical sense and hopefully still retain your sense of humour. I'll start this off with a personal evaluation which you can follow yourself.

After a shower, I'm having a good look in the full-length mirror. I see a fairly full head of grey hair, although I know that there is a growing patch of baldness at the back. At 65 kilograms and about 1.77 metres tall, I'm a little on the thin side, although in quite good shape courtesy of my daily exercise regime.

No double chins, although plenty of wrinkles, bags under my eyes, jowls forming either side of my chin and sundry spots on my face. Continuing on down, wrinkles continue, a reasonable chest, no big gut to speak of, and skinny, muscular legs and arms. A light tan completes the picture.

Summing up, genetics gifted me this slim body, and despite far too many beers and cigarettes over my earlier years, I am lucky, despite a few aches and pains, to be still healthy and able to live an active life.

Physically, that's it. Am I happy and fulfilled? Well, yes, Kate and I have a great life together, we have lots of connections to friends and family, and I still enjoy a stimulating, although now more relaxed, business life.

Now despite all this positivity, there are still dark moments; for example, you regularly lose people close to you as you grow older. You miss seeing them and hearing the sound of their voice. We are all going to have dark thoughts; it's how we deal with them that is the key.

Now take your own mental snapshot next time you take a shower. So what are you seeing in the mirror?

- Not bad for your age, or too soft and squishy, and room for improvement?
- What's your posture like? Upright and shoulders back or a bit stooped and listing to one side?
- Do you like what you see or are you a bit shocked by your appearance? The great thing here is, if you know how, there is always room for improvement.
- Get some inside info on your body to discover how incredible it is. Use your web browser to have a look at some of the Body World's images. When you look at one of these images, try to picture that under your skin, your own body is a miraculous structure.

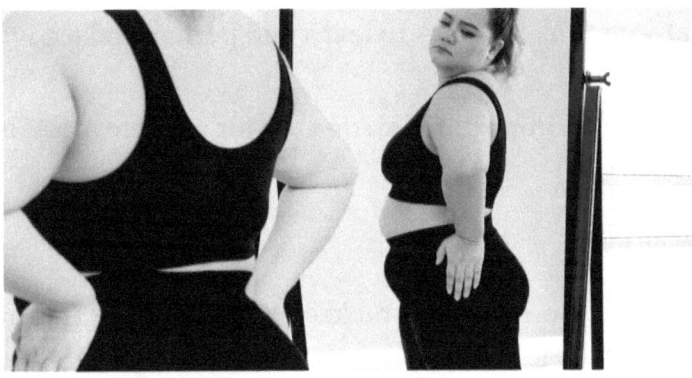

IMAGINING THE CHANGES

Your next step is to imagine how it would feel to be able to wind the clock back a few years and to regain some of the lost strength, agility and flexibility that you used to have. Also perhaps lose some weight and be able to fit into some of your old clothes. What would that be worth?

Well, this is entirely possible. You can incrementally improve all these things by making some simple food and lifestyle changes.

While I may have learned a lot about life and myself, and can write about all this, I am just like you or anybody else, and I also have ongoing struggles and self-doubt. Life isn't easy. I think once you recognise this, accept that 'shit happens' and that you just have to deal with it, it somehow makes things easier.

Uncertain times like the Covid-19 pandemic are really unsettling. How is it that some people can seem to take most unsettling situations in their stride? Coming to mind is Virgin's Richard Branson. Despite many setbacks along the way, he always seems to remain optimistic and is proactively looking for solutions to move forward. He accepts the situation, knows that he cannot control it and will always look for ways to learn and perhaps take advantage of it in some way.

These are such important lessons too for us mere mortals.

STICK TO YOUR GUNS

Feeling positive about all this and keen to get started? It is important to note that, like Branson, there will be hiccups along the way. Despite your best efforts, you may suffer setbacks like an injury or unexpected illness. It is crucial to stick to your guns and get back to your new lifestyle as soon as possible.

Be wary of the old trap of starting off with massive enthusiasm and gradually slackening off as all of life's other challenges get in the way. Through thick and thin, you need to be staunch and stick to your guns.

Right, it's time now to get down to business. Are you ready to start putting together your new life's challenge?

Back to the overarching idea of all this, which is that you are only gifted this one opportunity at life, and just this one body. Be sure to make the most of it and look after your precious body and mind.

So you've looked in the mirror, taken stock, and know there is work to do. The following is one simple idea you could try to help get you off to a good start.

YOUR INCREDIBLE BODY

Get some inside info on your body to discover how incredible it is. Have a look online at some of the 'Body Worlds' images. Seeing this exhibition was a defining moment for me and was the motivation I needed to take up my life's challenge. This exhibition is quite incredible, as it literally lays bare all parts of our bodies. You can see all the bones, muscles, tendons, ligaments and internal organs. One exhibit even showed the nerves in the brain, seemingly suspended in mid-air with all the other parts of it stripped away.

I formerly studied in the 'bod' room at medical school as part of my physical education training. (I can still remember the awful cloying smell of the formaldehyde.) The cadavers were inanimate objects, quite unlike the strikingly lifelike exhibits of the Body World. I can tell you, this exhibition changed the way I viewed my body, and now I fully appreciate what I've got. Sometimes I can even picture some of the actions of the muscles and tendons when I'm exercising. It is like 'getting under your skin' in the most positive way.

When you look at one of these exhibits, try to picture that under your skin, your own body has this same miraculous structure. Likewise for any movement you might make. Standing up, for instance, requires an incredible coordination of your quadriceps, gluteals and other muscles and ligaments, along with a complicated set of manoeuvres required from your brain, central nervous system, inner ear and more.

GRATITUDE

Another important idea in taking on this challenge of getting the best out of the rest of your life is to be grateful for this gift. How could you possibly just take it for granted or, worse still, neglect it? You could say that you are embarking on the ultimate goal.

Your challenge can take any shape you like and will of course reflect your various strengths and weaknesses.

The rest of this book is about helping to motivate you to take up your challenge and providing insights and tools to help you succeed.

I would first like to introduce you to Irene. I have compiled this story about Irene based on my experiences with so many people like her who passed through our rest home. I also received many referrals from medical practices of patients with equally sad stories.

IRENE'S STORY

 Irene is seventy-five years old and has lived in a rest home for the past three years. She can only walk now with the aid of a walker and at a very slow pace. She is frail, stooped over and has poor balance and is generally very weak physically. Her medical conditions include high blood pressure, type 2 diabetes, depression, neuropathy and atrial fibrillation. She is also incontinent and suffers from sleep apnoea.

Irene often reflects on her life.

'My daily routine now hardly ever varies. The nurse wakes me every morning at about 7.30 am, and the circus of getting me ready for breakfast begins.

'I have one of those fancy beds where the end raises up so they can get me out of bed easier. After a fair bit of manoeuvring, I am standing up holding onto my walker. Aches and pains everywhere, I'm just so stiff and sore these days.

'Off we trundle to the shower room which also includes a raised toilet. I am helped into my shower chair and my very kind and patient nurse showers, dries and dresses me and I am escorted down the hall to the breakfast room.

'I must say, mealtimes are a highlight and in the morning I can smell the bacon, coffee and other delicious aromas wafting around as I am helped into my chair.

'After breakfast, I am able to laboriously 'walker' my way into the adjacent lounge and watch TV for a while. As you can imagine, being as incapacitated now as I am, all the rest of my days follow similar patterns. Although it is frightfully boring and repetitive, I feel blessed that I am being looked after in this warm, safe and caring environment. I simply could not live independently now, and the thought of doing this really frightens me.

'Back in my room, I am propped up in bed by my carer so that I can read. Despite our cleaners' best efforts, I know my room smells; I only know this because my family tell me so. I must have got used to it.

'I often think back to when I was fit and well, playing regular golf and bowls, taking brisk daily walks and just loving my little garden.

'The doctor had told me a number of times that I needed to start blood pressure medication. I didn't listen, and at age sixty had a stroke which could well have been prevented.

'I lost some functions on my left side and my hospital physio did a wonderful job getting me mobile again. My GP told me that I had been really lucky and encouraged me to get back to my former active lifestyle.

'This is where I made my second big mistake. I thought I would just take it easy for a while and started watching lots of daytime TV and even got out my knitting again. Oh, how relaxing and easy my life now seemed.

'After having three children, I often had a bit of a problem with incontinence. A few years later the condition deteriorated, and my GP told me that I had a prolapse and a hysterectomy would help to sort this out. In the end, I took the soft option and had a pessary inserted to improve this problem. She warned me that this was probably only going to be a temporary measure. Did I listen?

'Over the next couple of years, I found it increasingly difficult to get out of my own way. My formerly active lifestyle had become sedentary.

Looking back on it, no wonder I got depressed. My daughters would come around and we would go out on little walks. Little, I say, as after a short time I would run out of breath and energy.

'Well, the rest is history. Over those next few years, only seven in total, I had many opportunities to turn things around, by slowly getting back to my former active lifestyle. It was as if I had lost touch with the reality of life and gradually I was losing all my independence. The family even had to get a gardener in, and one day, quite bewilderingly, I was told by a health assessor that I would have to go into a rest home.

'And now after three long years in the rest home I have lost all my dignity, am racked with pain in many places and have completely lost any independence or hope for a fulfilling life. At age seventy, I have had enough; I don't want to endure this any longer.

'The absolutely worst moments of my life now happen when I am visited by Carol and Judy, my ever-loyal former golfing and walking buddies. They both look so fit and well. Although they don't talk about their still-active lifestyles, for fear of upsetting me, I still get this feeling of overwhelming sadness at what I have missed out on.

'I am fearful and stressed about what my future holds for me, although welcome oblivion could not come quick enough.'

A cautionary tale indeed and one I have sadly heard too many times. Irene was a victim of death denial and did not listen to her GP's blood-pressure medication suggestion. After her stroke, she did not take advantage of what was really a major let-off for her and failed to get back to her former active lifestyle. Within a relatively short space of time, sadly her healthspan years were over.

3
CELEBRATE MOVEMENT

KEY POINTS

- The gift of movement is so often just taken for granted, yet even standing up requires a complex set of actions to occur.
- Imagine for a moment having this precious gift taken away.
- A lack of fitness is a major predictor of death and the contracting of chronic diseases. Regular exercise decreases the risk of diseases like heart, diabetes, cancer, osteoporosis and Alzheimer's.
- An important motivational aspect is that all movement counts towards improving your fitness, even household and gardening chores. It can be a game changer.
- You are far more likely to be able to continue to enjoy freedom of movement if you do indeed celebrate

movement and take every opportunity to do this. Make any movement an opportunity, not an imposition.

- How do you acquire the right frame of mind to celebrate all movement? First acknowledge how incredible your body is in allowing you to perform all the functions that you need to stay alive, enjoy life and have freedom of movement.
- Always be aware of the negative health aspects of long periods of sitting. Break these up with some form of exercise which will ideally get you puffing.
- Regular movement and exercise are key: every day, as often as you can, get moving and don't forget to celebrate that you can still do it.

THE GIFT OF MOVEMENT

The gift of movement is so often just taken for granted. A first step in understanding the significance of this is to get a handle on just how miraculous it is.

Even standing up requires a complex set of actions. Your skeleton allows you to maintain an upright position. To be able to stand up, your eyes, ears, brain, spinal cord, heart and muscles all need to work together to help you to do this seemingly simple action that we all take for granted.

Your eyes help you to stay upright by being able to see what's going on in the environment around us.

You may also have heard the expression, 'having rocks in your head',. Well, you really do. In your ears there are little calcium carbonate crystals which roll around in a fluid medium, which sends a signal to your nerves, which in turn sends a message to your muscles to tell them how to keep you upright.

Whenever we stand up, even your heart gets into the action by speeding up to counter the drop in blood pressure caused by this action. There are also special detectors in the muscles of your leg which will cause the muscles to contract to help you to maintain balance. And, of course, your brain and spinal cord mastermind all of this by continually sending messages to initiate the appropriate actions to all parts of your body.

This explains why stroke and spinal cord injuries so severely handicap people suffering from these issues. Because some of these pathways have been damaged, many people who are fortunate enough to have recovered, or partially recovered, often need to learn how to walk again.

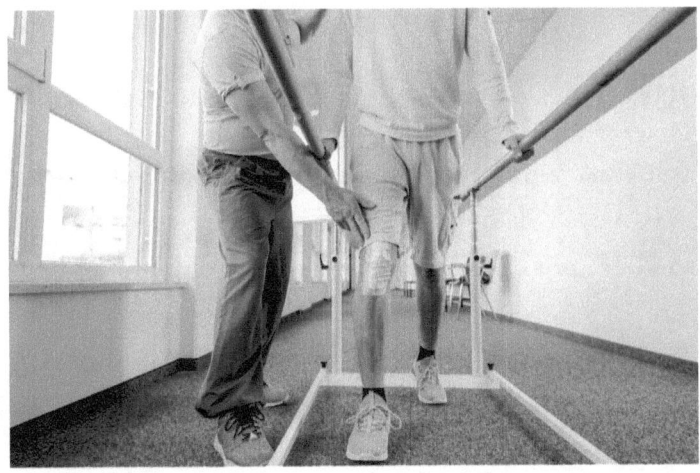

PROPRIOCEPTION

This need to learn to walk again can be partly explained by some of the person's proprioceptors, which are located in many parts of the body, going to sleep. These sensory receptors help us to make all of our different movements.

This overall concept is called proprioception, which is the ability to sense movement, action and location. In other words, the ability to move freely without consciously having to think about it. A simple example of this is to be able to walk without looking at your feet.

You will sometimes see older people walking hesitantly and looking down towards their feet. They may have lost function in this critical area.

People who have had long-term serious injuries to their legs sometimes need to learn to walk again because proprioceptors in their legs have gone to sleep and need to be reawakened.

The way to improve proprioception is of course to move more often. Any combinations of walking, dancing, lifting weights, skipping and many more possibilities for movement will all help.

MADE FOR MOVEMENT

Now, imagine for a moment having this precious gift of movement being taken away. This book is about helping to motivate you to give yourself the best possible chance, barring accidents, of never having this happen.

Even in the womb you were active, and your mother will attest to this after being subjected to many, many kicks over the last few months of pregnancy.

We are classified as upright terrestrials. Early men and women, who had to hunt and forage for food, despite having relatively short lives, were a seriously fit, lean and healthy lot by comparison with their modern counterparts.

The words in the title of the song 'These Boots Were Made for

Walking', are highly relevant. Whether or not you are barefoot or have boots, shoes or jandals on, those things at the end of your legs are built to walk, run, skip, jump, dance and ski; they play a crucial part in any other form of movement.

In modern society today, everything we need is conveniently gathered and packaged for us, and all our sundry devices like washing machines and clothes dryers have helped us to become less physically active. Also, all of those smaller devices, which so many of us are addicted to, have made our sitting times increase exponentially, making us even more sedentary.

Long periods of sitting are common and cause your metabolism to slow and calorie burning to decrease. A regular pattern of this can cause muscle wasting and risk of weight gain and diabetes.

FITNESS AND HEALTH

Fitness is the biggest predictor of death and the contracting of chronic diseases. Regular exercise decreases the risk of diseases like heart, diabetes, cancer, osteoporosis and Alzheimer's. Most of us know this stuff anyway, and keeping fit is really a no-brainer.

An important motivational aspect is that *all movement counts in improving your fitness, even household and gardening chores.* Studies have clearly proved this, and one in particular caught my attention. Harvard's Ellen Langer found that hotel maids easily exceeded the national requirement for exercise. Strangely, most of them did not think that they were fit. She split them into two groups with one carrying on as normal, while the other group were schooled by being told about the benefits of the various housekeeping activities they were doing each day.

At the end of the study, the group that had been schooled had lost weight and had other improvements in medical markers, like blood pressure levels, while the other group had stayed the same.

This was a game changer for this enlightened group, and another massive benefit for them was that they were now far more likely to enjoy their work, after understanding the benefits to their health and fitness.

Likewise, for anyone it can be a game changer if you can get a clear picture of the health benefits of any movement that you make.

MAKE ANY MOVEMENT AN OPPORTUNITY

We are lucky to enjoy freedom of movement, and this can be taken away from us in an instant; any paraplegic or stroke victim can attest to that.

So here's the thing: from a health perspective, you are far more likely to be able to continue to enjoy freedom of movement if you do indeed celebrate movement, and if you take every available opportunity to do this. *Make any movement an opportunity, not an imposition.*

As I write this, it's a beautiful sunny day. I've had an hour's walk on fairly hilly country this morning and a short cross-training session earlier this afternoon. Despite this, I still contemplate getting out there for a bit of a walk to earn my evening drink. After so many years of being like this, I'm hard wired for it. At the same time, I believe that it's never too late for anyone to acquire this habit, to whatever degree they are comfortable with. It can be positively life changing.

I also acknowledge that, thankfully, we are all different and that many people would rather curl up with a book than go for a brisk walk.

CELEBRATING ALL MOVEMENT

So how do you acquire the right frame of mind to celebrate all movement? First, it's as simple as first acknowledging how incredible your body is in allowing you to perform all of the functions that you need to stay alive, enjoy your life and have freedom of movement.

Second, get a clear picture that all movement helps you to become fitter no matter what it is. Gardening, housework, picking the mail up at the gate, walking the dog and obviously any form of dedicated exercise all help. The pictures you need to have in your mind are of the many health benefits that you are going to gain from this.

DOWN WITH SITTING

It also helps to be always aware of the negative health aspects of long periods of sitting. Break these up with some form of exercise that will ideally get you puffing. Tune yourself into listening to your body when exercising. Feel your heart beating faster and the blood flow increasing to all parts of your body. Celebrate all the coordinated movement that your legs and arms are making to help you walk or cycle up that hill. It's brilliant!

REGULAR MOVEMENT AND EXERCISE

Finally, regular movement and exercise are key; every day as often as you can, get moving and don't forget to celebrate that you can still do it.

In our next chapter we look at many different forms of

movement and exercise and their relevance to having a healthy and productive life.

PAT'S STORY

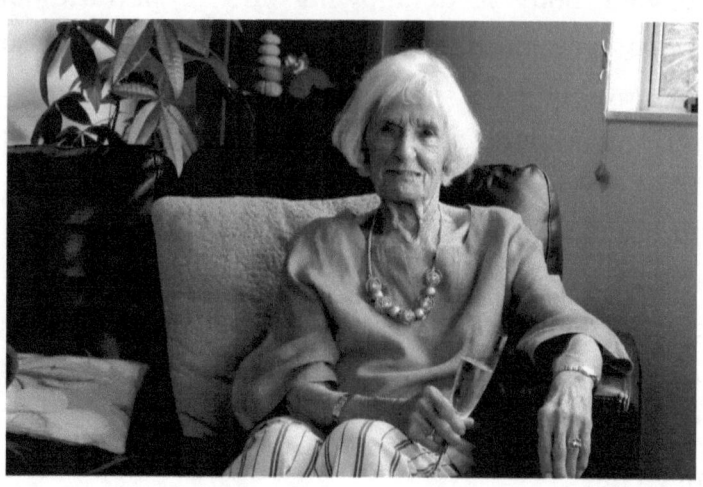

 Over the past two years I have met Pat around our retirement village and have shared some great stories over a couple of drinks.

What has always struck me about Pat is how quickly she moves; 'bright eyed and bushy tailed' sums her up perfectly.

A group of weary travellers straggled their way through our village lounge one night just before we were about to start a bingo night. Turns out they had been up north to Whangārei to see the fabulous Hundertwasser Art Centre.

The bus had been an hour late picking them up in the morning and some eight long hours later this tired group had arrived back. As they came through the lounge, I told the group that bingo was about to start.

They weren't having a bar of any bingo and were all making a beeline for their respective apartments. This was until I spotted Pat and her friend, who immediately brightened up at the prospect of having a crack at bingo. Within minutes they had drinks in hand and, clutching their bingo books, were off to find a seat.

I only found out recently that Pat is in her ninetieth year, and I marvel at the terrific energy she has and her great zest for life.

She was born in Liverpool in 1933, and she has told me that being a port town the war was horrendous, with Liverpool the most heavily bombed area outside London. They lived in an elevated position and saw it all happening before their eyes.

The children were put to bed in a reinforced cellar and listened to bombs falling all over the place. I can only imagine the terrible noises and the smoke, sirens and general chaos. They were lucky as two streets down houses were razed to the ground.

She and her sister were evacuated quite nearby down the coast. Her dad was a compulsive gambler and they never owned a house of their own. It was an unsettling life with many shifts. Despite this lack of any continuity with their education, Pat said they did well. She worked in an insurance company and her sister as a dental nurse.

Along the way she met her husband to be, Alan. He

was a Roman Catholic and because of the bigotry of that age, a favourite uncle never spoke to her again. There was similar fallout with other family and friends.

In 1961 Helen was born, and Kate followed two years later. Helen was slim like Pat and all she wanted to do was dress well and travel. On the other hand, Kate was well proportioned and very bright and studious.

The two girls married and Kate and her husband Steve, a sea captain, always wanted to live abroad and New Zealand was the country they settled on.

Pat said, 'Ooh, we like this place,' and after a number of visits, and some resistance from Alan, in 2002 they moved permanently to Auckland.

Pat and Alan had an adventurous life and travelled Europe in a campervan for three years and lived periodically in France. Helen had married a Frenchman called Guille and their family loved having Pat and Alan so close by.

Helen tragically died suddenly of an aneurysm in 2016. The last words spoken by Pat to Helen before she died were, 'We'll be here to help you, Helen,' and Helen had replied, 'Thanks, Mum.'

Guille and the grandchildren continued to stay close, and Pat has a huge regard for Guille. One day he said to her, 'Okay, Grandma, it's time we got you a computer.' And he got Pat up and running on the internet and she is grateful to this day for that kind gesture.

Over his life Alan had had some anxiety and depression issues, and he developed prostate cancer. At this stage they were living in a beautiful high-rise apartment, at Devon Towers in Devonport in Auckland.

After a while Pat found it hard to manage and had to call in nursing help for Alan's day-to-day health requirements. Eventually, Pat moved into a serviced apartment at the village where she now lives and Alan was sadly put into care. In 2002 Alan passed away and Pat moved into her own independent apartment which has beautiful harbour views.

Pat has found it hard to adjust to this way of life without Alan. She realised that she just needed to get on with it.

She says, 'I was born to walk quickly and Alan and I walked and sailed to our hearts' content.' Pat now walks regularly with Kate and her two dogs, attends exercise classes and is known to do little dances to music in her apartment. She says she always parks her car away from her intended destination to give herself a little walk.

Pat tells me that she knows a couple who have both climbed Everest. She muses that she has never done anything like this, and in fact has led a fairly ordinary life.

Well, Pat, while you have never physically climbed the tallest peak in the world you still have had your own Everest to climb.

Suffering the deaths of two of the dearest people in

your life could have been life changing. While you have grieved these losses, you have also managed to rebuild your life in a very positive way. No small feat.

Pat sums her life up:

'Food and wine are a must in my life to share with family and friends. These range from luxury restaurants to simple things like just having fish and chips on the beach.

'When I had Covid I realised what great neighbours I had. We all lost part of our lives during Covid and somehow we have bounced back.

'My independence means a lot to me, and my art, sewing, knitting, active lifestyle and kind people around me give me hope for the future.

'Although I certainly won't go down in history, on reflection I have got great excitement and enjoyment out of my life. And I'm still going!

'Being born a Liverpool North girl gave me attitude, a sense of humour and my feet on the ground.'

4
IN SEARCH OF HAPPINESS

KEY POINTS

- **Choice** – Apart from really extreme situations, such as living in war zones, most of us have options available to change our personal situations. It is up to you!
- **Attitude** – Satisfying the four pillars for having the right attitude to life is crucial to being happy. You have to get these criteria right first.
- **Serenity, courage and wisdom** – I just love Niebuhr's prayer in relation to being serene about what you can't change, being courageous about changing the things you can and having the wisdom to know the difference.
- **Acceptance** – I believe this prayer leads us on to being grateful and accepting.
- Many people would benefit from a daily dose of focusing on the positive aspects of their lives.

- **FOMO (fear of missing out) vs JOMO (joy of missing out)** –Finding a balance between the two would make for a calmer and more contented existence. And a happier life.
- We simply cannot be happy all of the time. We need to make our periods of happiness just that much longer.

CHOOSING HOW WE LIVE

Achieving the state of happiness always seems to be elusive. When I started writing this book, I did not intend including a chapter on this subject. On reflection I have changed my mind after deciding that being happy is such a basic element in getting the best out of the rest of your life.

The definition of being happy is to be in a state where you are experiencing positive emotions like joy, fulfilment, satisfaction and contentment.

And sadness will obviously be the opposite and encompass negative emotions.

Inevitably, fate will play an enormous part in whether or not you are happy or sad. People who live in areas ravaged by violence, famine or war are facing terrible hardship and grief.

Some people will be able to rise above it all and wring whatever drop of happiness they can out of their perilous lives.

Regardless of any of our different life situations, we all have some choice as to how we will live it.

Obviously, people in these seriously compromised living conditions and danger have far fewer options than others in more affluent and settled countries.

I always find it so sad to hear about someone taking their own life. This is more amplified when you know that person. In my family's case, we experienced two suicides in a little more than a year. When I was fourteen years old, my brother took his own life on the eve of my sister's wedding.

You can only imagine the chaos and grief which followed after poor Mum found my brother Dale hanging in our garage on the morning of the wedding.

A year later, my father also took his own life on the corner of Cashel and Manchester Streets, Christchurch by throwing himself in front of a truck.

I had always been told by my family that this had been an accident. I found out some fifty years later that he had actually taken his own life. Phil, a nephew of mine who is a researcher, intrigued by his family's history, found the coroner's report. There it was in black and white, the two witnesses' statements, brutally confirming that it had been no accident.

Throughout history all families will have the saddest things happen, and like ours, sometimes multiple tragedies. This was our family's turn.

A neighbour of ours once told me one day that after the death of my brother Dale she never again heard my mother singing while she hung out the clothes. My mum Essie was a wonderfully happy and outgoing person, who did sing while she hung out the washing and would often go dancing and partying.

Although to me she remained that happy person, deep down she must have suffered some terrible grief.

Essie had a choice between dwelling on what must have been many negative emotions or trying to stay positive and to get on with life the best way possible. She obviously chose the latter.

THE IMPORTANCE OF GAINING CLARITY

Our modern world provides us with many different choices for education, travel, sport and leisure. And our access to so many different tech devices opens up a world of infinite possibilities.

All this proliferation can cause confusion and uncertainty as to what the best options might be.

I think to be happy you need to gain some clarity as to what the parameters of your life are going to be. Otherwise, it will be very difficult to be contented and satisfied if you are always second guessing what you should be doing.

Some of the happiest people I have ever seen are people with handicaps which narrow down both their life and employment options. I have seen a number of segments on current affairs TV programmes that have kept track of staff of companies who largely employ handicapped people.

Their roles are generally repetitive tasks like cleaning, packaging products or stacking shelves. They have a purpose in life and take real pride in their work and have great relationships with their colleagues and the business managers. This just shines out of them when you see their happy smiles and positive body language during these programmes.

By way of genetics or disease or accident, their options in life have been limited. They certainly know how to seize the day and are grateful for and make the very best out of what they've got.

I just love seeing these programmes.

A HAPPINESS INDEX

I thought it would be interesting to use a happiness index in all of the key areas of your life. How would you rate your own level of happiness out of ten?

The key areas are your relationship with your spouse or partner, your job, financial situation, health, social life and leisure and sporting activities.

You need to be realistic. It is much easier for me as a retired person in good health and with reasonable financial means to be happy. No mortgages, dependent children or job makes for a pretty uncluttered and relaxed lifestyle.

Married with children, with a mortgage and both partners working makes for a hectic life. Juggling all of the competing priorities that get thrown at you daily is hard work.

With six areas your highest possible score is sixty. At the moment, I score quite highly. Now take away my good health and the game changes dramatically. If your healthspan years end because of one debilitating illness or other, your happiness index would take a big hit.

Relationships with our partner or spouse are also a huge factor. Domestic violence levels remain high and you read of these horrendous situations that mainly woman seem to face.

If you and your children are facing physical and mental abuse on a day-to-day basis, there is no chance that you are going to be happy. Every waking moment is probably spent trying to keep the peace and fearing for your and your children's future.

Once again it all comes back to choice. If you are in one of these situations, you have two choices – to stay or to leave. There are many established Women's Refuge centres and our police and other agencies are very familiar and experienced with these situations. A well thought--out plan can be hatched to safely extricate families from these atrocious situations.

The day you leave is day one of your new life. Every day that you stay prolongs your uncertain and potentially dangerous life.

The same applies for anyone. The papers are full of sad stories about young children and adults suffering from life-threatening diseases like cancer. I am amazed at the courage and tenacity these individuals and families display during these really tough times. Sometimes children spend years in hospital and the parents somehow adapt their lives to meet these new challenges.

Despite the toll and grind of these seemingly endless medical procedures, these families dig in and make the very best of these tough situations. You can see the love for each other shining through whenever the media cover their stories. Despite other aspects of their lives being put on hold, they must feel proud of their efforts and happy that they have left no stone unturned in seeking a positive health result.

Through no fault of their own their choices have become narrowed down to this one life or death goal. If they can get through this huge challenge and their loved one is saved, they will appreciate life far more and be one very happy family.

We now live in a chaotic world where the only certainty in life is change. Social media dominates so many people's lives. Their ability to spend quality time socialising face to face diminishes in this arm's-length, facile type of existence. They flit from sound bite to sound bite on TikTok, Instagram, Facebook and other platforms all eager to draw them into their spider webs.

No question, social media used in moderation is highly entertaining and a brilliant way of interacting with your family and friends. Once again, it all comes down to choice as to whether you can reach a healthy balance.

THE FOUR PILLARS

Inevitably, my random dissertation on being happy comes back to the basics of having the right attitude. To me these criteria are the four pillars which happiness sits on: *being positive, socially engaged, challenged and having a purpose in life.*

To score highly on this happiness index I believe you need to satisfy all of these criteria. My only question would be the one about being well connected. I know people you would class as loners, and their utopia is life in a log cabin in a remote spot in the mountains.

Likewise, there will always be people who will break the mould and be exceptions to our attitude criteria.

Searching vs serenity

Another key disrupter to happiness is to be continually searching for something. This can come in many forms, as in 'keeping up with the Joneses'. I must have a fancy new lawnmower just like our neighbours.

A scary new fad seems to be the widespread interest in surgical procedures which replace, repair or reconstruct parts of the body. Collectively known as plastic surgery or cosmetic surgery, all these tucks, trims and lifts banish wrinkles and prop up sagging body parts. You name it: chins, cheeks, lips, breasts, tummies and more get this ultimate primping treatment.

Some such surgery makes medical sense, but many are not without unfortunate or uncomfortable side-effects.

Rolling the dice indeed!

This brings me to the well-known Serenity Prayer, the original of which is attributed to the influential American theologian Reinhold Niebuhr in the 1930s:

'God, grant me the serenity to accept the things that I cannot change, courage to change the things that I can, and wisdom to know the difference.'

All it takes is serenity, courage and wisdom. Easier said than done, and so relevant to these tricky decisions people have to make on elective surgery.

And this also applies to so many other aspects of our lives.

FOMO VS JOMO

FOMO is the fear of missing out; JOMO is the joy of missing out. These two acronyms stand in direct opposition to each other and, I believe in their own way, are very important concepts in finding happiness. *Striking a balance between the two can make a huge difference.*

Our modern lives today can be a chaotic hubbub, chock full of clutter and competing priorities and opportunities, tailor-made for rampant FOMO behaviour.

We now deal in enormous quantities of information. We scroll through screeds of pieces of info on our phones and other devices, quickly sifting out bits we like and discarding others.

Even though these days I have plenty of time, I too follow this same pattern to read newspapers and social media feeds. It is the nature of the beast; there is just so much available info being hurled at us on so many platforms.

Among all of this clutter inevitably come myriad opportunities to do things. It can be invitations to everything from product launches to a once in a lifetime opportunity to view a blue moon eclipse. Movies, birthdays, weddings, fishing trips and more are also on the list. It's all on for young and old.

Social media provides access at the touch of a button to this amazing all-encompassing landscape of opportunity.

There is just so much stuff. Competing priorities and images continually flash in front of you of people having a wonderful time and this may lead to an uneasy feeling that you just might be missing out.

'Scarcity' is a basic concept of economics. It's the gap between limited supply and greater demand. This is a beautiful thing for businesses with a product which is immensely popular. Not so much for many consumers, particularly those with a FOMO bent.

Crowded House sold out the Sydney Opera house for one of their concerts in just a few minutes. This happens everywhere and any time that something or someone is immensely popular but the supply of a product or service is limited.

Fortunately, the antidote to avoid continually being in this awful FOMO state is a good dose of JOMO. The joy of missing out is the opposite state, where people are happy and contented in their own space, and grateful for what they have got.

Looking back, I've certainly been a FOMO candidate in my younger years. Out on the water fishing with not much happening, you become sure that that boat over there has been catching more than you. And so up anchor and motor over their way, perhaps to only experience the same lack of bites again.

Missing out on being picked for teams or invites to parties, and feeling a bit left out at times socially come to mind. I'm sure there have been plenty of other long-forgotten FOMO episodes.

This is an important point. When tomorrow comes, a new day

beckons with new opportunities and yesterday's disappointments are forgotten.

I am far more often these days in JOMO mode than I was when I was younger. I think this is a natural ageing thing where your boundaries naturally diminish a bit. It was not too long ago that attending All Blacks rugby tests was a must. These days I'm very contented sitting on my couch in the warm, with beer and chips handy and feeling a bit smug about all those punters out there in the freezing cold.

5
HAVING THE RIGHT ATTITUDE

KEY POINTS

- Having the right attitude includes being positive and socially engaged as well as having a sense of purpose and being challenged. This attitude can help people prevent the diseases of old age.
- **Are you ready?** In all my twenty years of helping people with weight, diabetes and other lifestyle issues, there was always one common theme: people who were ready to commit to making a few permanent changes to their lifestyle always succeeded.
- Once you know you are ready, a few simple concepts may help you to succeed:
  - **Reviewing** your exercise habits and regime, including using open-ended questions, which force you to find solutions.

- **Being positive** —The first step to staying positive is to not worry about things you can't control and focus on things that you can.
- **Always go glass half full** or partly sunny day.
- **Being socially engaged** – The Grant Study found strong relationships to be far and away the strongest predictor of life satisfaction and better predictors of long and happy lives than social class, wealth, fame, IQ, or even genes.
- **Having a purpose and being challenged** – Getting through your working life and bringing up families provide their own natural purposes and challenges. Your retirement years are a different story, and a lack of purpose can lead to a fairly hollow existence.

A DIY APPROACH TO HEALTHCARE

Harry de Quetteville, writing in the UK's *Daily Telegraph* on 4 October 2022, says that a key part of UK doctor Sir Muir Gray's definition of having the right attitude is 'Being positive and socially engaged and having a sense of purpose and being challenged.'

Sir Muir is a visionary Scottish doctor who has made significant inroads into improving public health outcomes in the UK. This includes pioneering their NHS disease-screening programme, and more recently, the Dementia Risk Reduction Programme.

He tells this very personal story of someone young: his daughter Tat. Now in her thirties, she developed type 1 diabetes in her teens and then broke her back skiing. It led, says Sir Muir, to a decade of pain, to '10 years of problems not being resolved medically until she decided "this can't go on" and went to a gym and sorted herself out'.

Gray thinks that the message of self-reliance has ramifications far beyond Tat. 'Healthcare is what you do for yourself,' he says. 'It is the most important care, followed by informal care by friends, family and volunteers. Then comes professional care.'

It is a DIY attitude, he says, that can help people prevent the diseases of old age ruining their lives or even getting a grip in the first place. This attitude focuses on maintaining or recovering strength, stamina, suppleness and sociability whose loss many of us assume is an inevitable consequence of ageing. It thus reduces the period of serious debility to as soon as possible before death.

Not that Gray, who spent many years at the top of the NHS, dismisses the brilliance or necessity of doctors and medicine. It's simply that 'over the last forty years, the health service has become a bit focused only on drugs and technology'. And as it has done so, he thinks, 'we patients have become passive about our own health, particularly when it comes to dementia'.

ARE YOU READY?

In all my twenty years of helping people with weight, diabetes and other lifestyle issues, there was always one common theme: *clients who were ready always gained benefits, with some of these being life changing.* What do I mean by ready? It is having the ability to make a few simple and permanent changes to their lifestyle.

About half the people who learned our concepts gained benefits. Some of these were small like modest weight loss, and others were life changing. Losing fifty to sixty kilograms, reversing a type 2 diabetes condition, reducing blood pressure and improving other medical markers were in this category.

There was one other common theme. After a short time, the

other half who were doomed to failure would always be making excuses. Been away, had a cold, had relatives staying and many other variations on these.

On the other hand, those that succeeded would find ways to do so by making their lifestyle changes permanent through thick and thin. No matter what was thrown at them. *They were ready!*

If you have decided to take up your challenge of trying to get the best out of the rest of your life, you first need to be ready. Once you know you are ready, a couple of simple concepts may help you to succeed.

REVIEWING

You may have already written down some of the lifestyle things that you are going to change and need to keep these at front of mind. A daily review is a great way to do this.

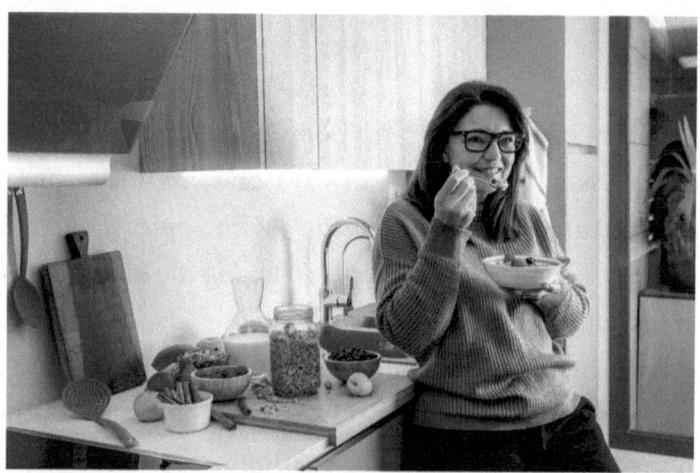

Ideally, you should find a few minutes each day to review. Often, our busy lives just get in the way, and before you know it your day is over, and other priorities like preparing the evening meal take over.

I find the best way to find a few moments is to do a quick review while you are eating your lunch or over your afternoon coffee.

Another good time is just before you go off to sleep.

Open-ended questions

This sort of calm review is similar to what is widely known as mindfulness. The rules are simple: be present in the moment and take a non-judgemental view. In other words, focus completely on your review and don't beat yourself up over anything.

Open or open-ended questions force you to come up with both answers and solutions: 'How did my exercise regime go today?' If the answer is negative, the next question can be, 'What am I going to do to put this right?'

Your answer might be to make sure you put your gear in your car tomorrow.

Open-ended questions are powerful agents and are at the heart of life coaching. This is where coaches are getting their clients to work through issues and discover solutions. I used these all the time with my clients when I was a coach. I now use them effectively in my day-to-day life working through various issues and problems.

Give it a go; although it takes a bit of practice, this method can positively change your life.

BEING PREPARED

Being prepared is my second useful concept. If you are trying to establish a new habit like having regular reviews or setting up a daily exercise programme, you need to get organised.

Think about what you want to achieve the next day and make sure you have set aside the time and have the right gear on hand. Once again, it's an open-ended question. 'What have I got on tomorrow?' and 'What do I need to get organised for this?'

Sounds too easy? Well, it is easy, and you will be surprised at how effective this simple stuff is in helping you to get organised and solving problems.

JUNE'S STORY

Now before we get back to Sir Muir's concept of having the right attitude, I would like to introduce you to June. I met June shortly after Kate and I had moved into our new retirement village. And what a privilege knowing her has been.

At the time of writing, the queen had only just passed away and we had noted that June, at age ninety-seven, was one year older than the wonderful Elizabeth Regina.

We knew that June had been a successful singer, dancer and actor in the West End of London and we were keen to find out more about her earlier life, which must have been fascinating. One evening we organised a small group to get together in our bar with June to do this.

June had formerly lived in a town on England's south coast called Shoreham-by-Sea, which is not far from Brighton. When she was sixteen, and developing into an excellent singer, it was suggested that she should sing to the troops who were stationed nearby.

'Our town was full of troops waiting to head off to Germany. Poor chaps, away from their homes and the fear of war too.'

Her mother agreed that she could, although with the proviso that it would only be twice a week. I asked her whether she used to get cheers and great applause from the troops. June replied drily, 'If I was lucky.' We all thought that was rather funny.

'One time they asked me to sing a song called "Yours" five times. I think they must have been pulling my leg.'

This was of course typical of June being her modest self, and far from the truth of it.

I also asked her what the main reason for her success had been. Very succinctly she said, 'I had good legs.' We could see from the many brilliant old photos she had brought along that she was right. And we all laughed when I replied, 'We can all see that.'

Her father was a shoemaker and had been trained in the early 1900s. Once he had his own shop, nobody left before having had a good laugh.

'He was an amusing man and I adored him.'

June used to worry about his swimming habits. He used to rush home from work winter or summer and, togs on, would be off to the nearby beach.

He used to swim out a long way. He told June that if she was worried about how far out he was going, he would lie on his back and put his leg in the air. This was to presumably signal that he was okay.

When he was in his seventies, he started to feel the cold while swimming and became quite ill.

June said, 'It was with much pleasure and delight that Daddy came to live with me. He was so appreciative of every little thing that I did for him. My two sisters who lived in Canada used to say what trouble it must be looking after Dad.

'He lived with me for eight months before he passed away and it was all such a pleasure and delight.'

When June left school, she wanted to go to drama school. Her parents insisted that she go to a commercial college first. In hindsight this proved to be a godsend as there were times during her professional acting and singing career where she was out of work. The office temping jobs filled these gaps brilliantly.

Although her heart was in acting, because she was a good singer most of her work was in this field. She has a passion for Shakespeare, but sadly no parts came her way as the standard of acting in the area was so brilliant.

June came to New Zealand about forty years ago and Karen Kay became her new agent, and the two have remained great friends ever since.

'She was a very good agent and used to ring me and say she had a possible job. My first question would always be, how much?

'Nine times out of ten, I would audition and get the job. This was because she knew my strengths.'

I asked June if she remembered any particular job. One she recalled was for a filmed advertisement set in a rest home. A resident is sitting in her room and sees a pussy cat go by. She gets excited and, wanting to find out where the cat is going, follows it on her walker.

The camera crew are out in the corridor, and June, on her walker, is supposed to follow the cat. The cat wouldn't play ball and kept turning back towards her. It was evidently hilarious and everybody was laughing. Eventually, the cat supplier turned up with a couple of other kittens and finally they were able to finish the ad. June was around ninety-four at the time.

She thought it was quite funny when I pointed out that she hadn't quite retired after all. I wondered how many other people would be making ads at that age.

I asked her what some of the key things were that had allowed her to live such a long and healthy life. She told me that she had always kept fit and still had regular sessions in our pool. I knew that until a couple of years ago that she was often seen walking around the village.

Acting and dancing were very demanding physically with some really long hours involved.

Her weight had not varied much since she was young, and she thought she may even be a little lighter.

'I was always conscious of what my weight was and how I felt. I would watch my diet to that extent and never ate many sugary things. Nine stone four [59 kg] was about average, I think.

'I have always had a daily dose of cider vinegar mixed with honey, and, of course, my daily tipple of red wine.

'And you know, you always need to have a purpose and some passion in your life.'

June explained how she had a great passion for the music on our own radio Concert Programme and that she had daily contact with her two sons and regularly kept in touch with her friends.

I have been told so often by people I have known in their late eighties or nineties that most of their friends had gone. Living in a retirement village really helps to ease that sadness due to the opportunity to meet many people daily who also have had interesting lives.

On moving in to the William Sanders Village, June knew that things would never be quite the same. 'You just need to adapt, and the sooner the better.'

June thought that gratitude was one of the most important parts to anyone's life. It allowed you to focus on all the positive things that you have and enjoy, rather than any negative aspects of your life.

June was very excited about her family coming the following week from overseas for Christmas and her daughter is staying on for three months. She said delightedly, 'I won't even have to worry about food as they are all such good cooks.'

Well, June, what a splendid couple of hours we had with you. If I had to think of one word to sum you up, it would be 'stylish'. Always beautifully dressed and with stylish hair to match. Even your walking stick which you sometimes use looks like an artistic masterpiece with its rainbow colours and bright patterns.

Walking slowly and carefully these days, although still very upright, you gracefully acknowledge anybody who passes by.

You were the star attraction on this evening and we loved listening to your gentle, cultured voice and the colourful experiences and life you have had. I noted that, despite the great interest in all things, you were also really present while listening to anything we had to offer.

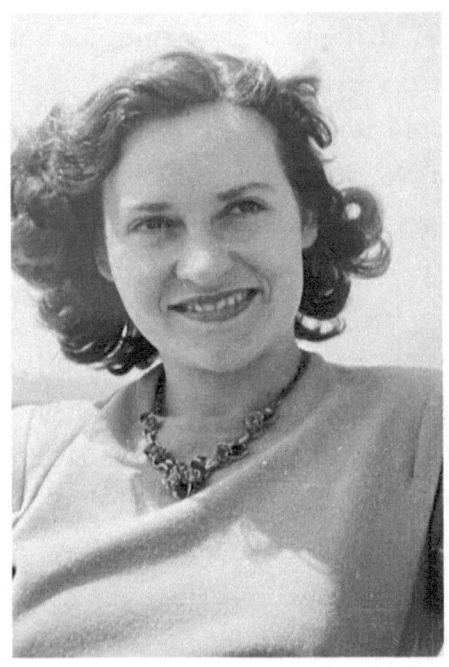
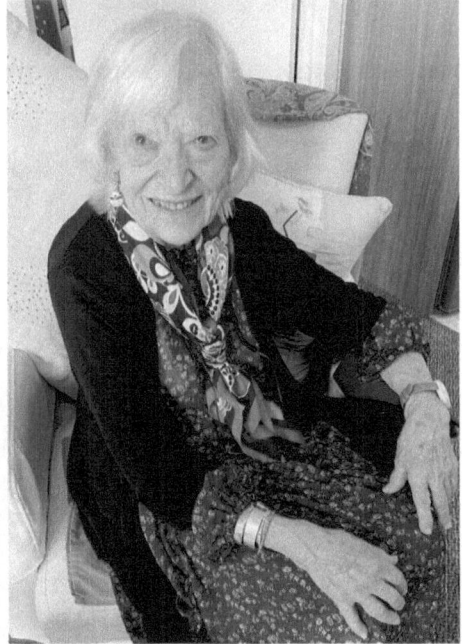

Now back to Sir Muir's definition of having the right attitude; how many boxes did June tick?

Being positive, socially engaged and having a purpose are the first three criteria that she can tick off. The fourth is to be challenged. My guess is that at age ninety-seven it would be challenge enough to live a normal and largely independent life as she still does so well.

Thanks, June, for sharing your life with us. At this stage she has a healthspan of ninety-seven years and is still counting. Absolutely fantastic!

We could even call her Shoreham-by-Sea's own Vera Lynn.

Time now to delve further into Sir Muir's criteria for having the right attitude.

POSITIVITY

It's all very well to say, 'stay positive'. Living in today's complex and sometimes confusing world is not easy.

No matter where you lived, Covid really tested all of us, and killed many of us. Even though, in New Zealand, we were locked down for long periods of time, I always felt grateful that we were not suffering the huge loss of life experienced by countries like the UK and America.

Right from the get-go we were constantly bombarded by shocking images. Bodies were being piled into mass graves, hospital wards overflowing with desperately ill people and many of the brave doctors and nurses sadly succumbing themselves.

Supply-chain hold-ups around the world stopped the flow of food, drink, medical supplies and every other commodity you could think of. Share markets tanked and people feared for their lives and their livelihoods.

I hate to think of the mental torture suffered by so many. Not able to attend loved ones' funerals and not even being able to see them on their last days.

People were separated from loved ones for months and sometimes years. Miraculously, vaccines were developed in record time and anti-viral drugs dramatically reduced the risk of dying.

Somehow the world has gradually recovered, and although Covid is now taking a back seat, the threats continue. Wars, riots, floods, wildfires, political turmoil, earthquakes, economic distress, staff shortages, tariff wars, mass murders, terrorism and the list just goes on.

FOCUS ON WHAT YOU CAN CONTROL

How do you stay positive? The first step is to not worry about things you can't control and focus on things that you can.

Well, you just can't control massive things like the climate, politics, wars or tax policies. Although we all need to show some interest in what's going on, the trick is not to get too emotionally caught up in it as you simply can't win.

Focus on what you can control. How much you spend, what you spend it on, your health, work–life balance, and more.

Once you have done everything possible to get something right, you must let go and see how things play out. Endlessly agonising over an outcome is both very tiring and a waste of time.

It is the human condition, and we all do it. The less you do it, the better your life will be. You have put your job application in and worked hard to get it right. You have done the same in a recent exam. Celebrate your effort and await the outcome. Endlessly fretting about these things that you can't control is hard going.

GLASS HALF FULL

Always go glass half full or 'partly sunny day'. I get so annoyed with weather forecasters saying, 'partly cloudy day', when the opposite is also true and sounds so much more positive.

Having said all that, we all know that our different personality types will largely dictate what our natural instincts will be. Some people are naturally pessimistic, and others are naturally optimistic. I tend to be an overly optimistic type and subsequently suffer a few disappointments as a result.

Ideally, we would recognise where we land in this area of our personality and be able to adjust accordingly.

SOCIALLY ENGAGED

Moving on to Sir Muir's next criterion for having the right attitude. The Grant Study, which has been running in America since 1942, provides compelling evidence that being socially engaged plays a massive part in your happiness and well-being.

It is a study of hundreds of American men, which includes both Harvard graduates and a large group of more underprivileged men. In 2021, the results were described:

The study found strong relationships to be far and away the strongest predictor of life satisfaction, and better predictors of long and happy lives than social class, wealth, fame, IQ, or even genes. That finding proved true across the board among both the Harvard men and the inner-city participants.

This eighty-year study surely is a ringing endorsement of the huge value of warm and loving relationships.

Having a close circle of friends and families who you regularly socialise with is gold. And WhatsApp, FaceTime and other platforms help us to easily connect with those who are living away from us.

If you live alone, it is even more important for you to have this close network around you. If you are in the unfortunate position of not having this support, it is really important to join local clubs and social groups to meet new people.

Retirement villages are the ultimate in providing close contact and the sharing of many different social activities with a wide range of people.

As with Kate and me, you find like-minded people to spend time with, while living fully independent lives ourselves.

If you are feeling lonely and in need of companionship, it is up to you to make the first move. And don't delay. Joining a local walking group or any other activity which you enjoy will immediately get you into the mix.

PURPOSE AND CHALLENGE

Having a purpose and being challenged are the final criteria.

Getting through your working life and bringing up families provides their own natural purposes and challenges. Your retirement years are a different story, and there are only so many games of golf and bridge that you can play in a week. While any competitive game like these two can provide a decent challenge, a lack of purpose can lead to a fairly hollow existence.

A purpose can be as simple as providing regular grandkid duties, which are good fun and really help out the parents. And you can hand them back.

Volunteering is also rewarding, and I love hearing about and seeing on TV great stories about people who are doing this. You can see the great enjoyment they get out of it and the love and respect you see being given back in spades by any recipients of their endeavours.

Like June, her passion for the Concert Programme is providing a purpose in life during her twilight years. She only has three years to go before bringing up her century. Her boundaries have reduced somewhat and her passion for music is just the ticket for helping to provide her with some real quality of life.

If you feel like you are just drifting rudderless through your life, it's time to take stock. Start volunteering, walk a dog or do whatever it takes for you to feel like you now have a purpose and a challenge in life to get you out of bed each morning.

Having the right attitude is a state of mind. If you are not happy with your attitude, you need to take some time out to think about it. This will help you to get your mind around it and make the necessary changes. In my experience, this could be positively life changing.

6

SPORT AND OTHER LEISURE ACTIVITIES

KEY POINTS

- **The benefits of walking:**
    - **Cardiovascular fitness** – Regular walks, particularly if they are brisk and involve some sort of hill climb, will improve your overall fitness.
    - **Mental health** – Brisk walking helps to release endorphins which will help you feel happier and more positive.
    - **Prevent osteoporosis** – Regular walking can help prevent osteoporosis by strengthening bones and muscles.
    - **Other benefits include** improving joint function, losing weight and giving you a longer life span than your non-walking counterparts.

- - **Physical functionality** – Walking will improve your chances of delaying deterioration in your physical functionality.
  - **Quality walks:** A gentle stroll for thirty minutes on flat terrain is obviously beneficial. These benefits are dramatically ramped up by moving at a more rapid pace up a hill. Greater intensity of walking increases your heart and breathing rate and creates more stress on your bones, joints, muscles and other soft tissues. This increased blood flow, oxygen uptake and other stresses provide benefits like raising your metabolic rate, reducing your blood sugar levels and helping to strengthen many of your body's tissues.

WALKING WONDERS

I have cherry picked a few activities which are universally popular and available and which provide considerable physical foundation-blocks benefits.

One such activity is walking. I cover this extensively as it is such a simple, accessible and enjoyable activity you can do anytime, anywhere.

One of the real joys of our lives are our daily walks. Thinking back, this was not always the case as most of my exercise used to come from a variety of activities like golf, tennis, biking, windsurfing and jogging. From age fifty, some of these former activities dropped away. Kate and I started walking regularly and always trying to seek out challenging and picturesque locations.

Fortunately, we lived in a beautiful deer farm park locality, with dramatic coastal scenery and no shortage of hilly, lung-busting climbs. And the local Whangārei Heads area provided us with other similar halcyon walks and beaches.

After selling our rest home in 2002, we moved to Mount Maunganui which also provided us with similar beautiful and challenging walks.

Over the years we developed the walking 'bug' and delight in getting our daily fix. Although I could never imagine a life without it now, I never take it for granted.

A daily walk can give you so many benefits. For us it is always a bit of an adventure. We mix up our walks by using different tracks and routes. We often run into people we know. This social aspect of it is often an unexpected bonus and provides a good opportunity to catch up, sometimes ending in a coffee stop at a local café.

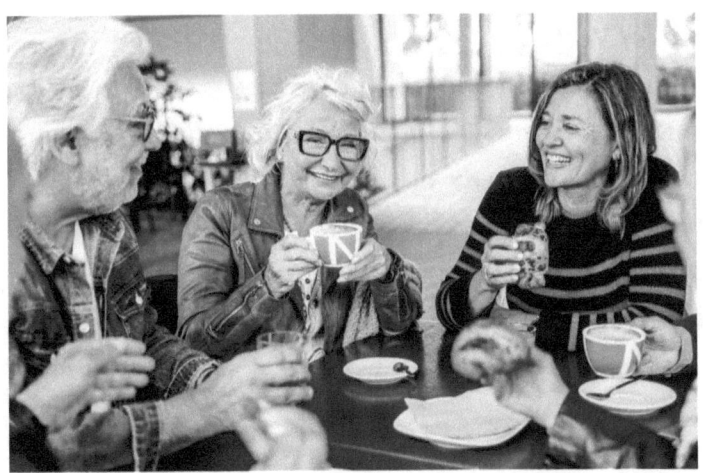

Nature always provides such an incredible backdrop. The change of seasons gives us the brilliant colours of autumn leaves and the contrasting new blossoms of spring, interspersed with the always fantastic and diverse range of greens. And if you're fortunate enough to be by the water, somewhere at the seaside, lake or river, the sound and sight of waves or other moving water can be quite hypnotic.

So, whether you are walking at a leisurely pace or puffing your way up a steep hill, it's a great opportunity to really engage your senses. Take in all the amazing sights, smells and sounds that are always there. I often pinch off a piece of lavender or rosemary and crush it in my fingers to smell the pungent aromas.

Alright, I know that I'm biased. Nonetheless, I'd highly recommend this simple, free and readily available activity to anyone who wants to change their life for the better.

The research on the benefits of daily walking is also compelling. I would like to thank the Arthritis Foundation of Georgia, USA for their permission to use this excellent following article from their website.

Benefits of Walking

What's not to like about walking? It's free. It's easy to do, and it's easy on the joints. And there's no question that walking is good for you. A University of Tennessee study found that women who walked had less body fat than those who didn't walk. It also lowers the risk of having blood clots. The calf acts as a venous pump, contracting and pumping blood from the feet and legs back to the heart, reducing the load on the heart. In addition to being an easy aerobic exercise, walking is good for you in many other ways.

Cardiovascular fitness – *Regular walks, particularly if they are brisk and involve some sort of hill climb, will improve your overall fitness.*

Increased heart rate and oxygen uptake will help to reduce your chance of having heart disease or stroke.

Prevent osteoporosis – *Regular walking can help prevent osteoporosis by actually strengthening both your bones and muscles.*

This is particularly relevant for post-menopausal women, and studies show that these regular walks can dramatically decrease the risk of hip fractures.

Look after your mental health
Brisk walking helps to release endorphins which will help you to feel happier and more positive.

This will also help to improve your sleep patterns and slow down memory decline in later life. These benefits could reduce your risk of dementia and Alzheimer's disease.

Other benefits include *improving joint function, losing weight and, according to research, having a longer life span than your non-walking counterparts.*

Physical functionality *– Improve your chances of not having failing physical functionality and delay this until later in life. This also reduces your chance of having any physical disability.*

WALKING QUALITY VERSUS QUANTITY

A gentle stroll for thirty minutes on flat terrain is obviously beneficial. These benefits are dramatically ramped up by moving at a more rapid pace uphill. Adding a faster pace or a hill or both increases the intensity of your walk.

This increases your heart and breathing rate and creates more stress on your bones, joints, muscles and other soft tissues. This increased blood flow, oxygen uptake and other stresses provide benefits like raising your metabolic rate, reducing your blood sugar levels and helping to strengthen many of your body's tissues. It also releases endorphins, those mood-enhancing hormones which can help reduce pain and stress and give you an overall sense of well-being.

Mixing in some higher intensity periods into your walks will help you to achieve some of these benefits.

DEVELOPING A WALKING PLAN

Despite now living in a lovely coastal setting with a fairly benign climate, I am constantly bemused by how few people we see out walking.

I believe that so many people are kept busy by the demands of their complex lifestyle, juggling work, family and other commitments, that taking regular walks seems like a bridge too far.

This is such a pity because this simple and free activity could be such a crucial factor in helping to substantially increase their vital healthspan years.

When I was working sixty-hour-plus weeks, I used to make an appointment in my diary each day to exercise. This worked really well for me. Otherwise, my busy days would have just disappeared, and I would have been too knackered at the end of it to even contemplate changing into my gear.

If you have read all my enthusiastic ramblings about how wonderful walking is and thinking, well, maybe you should give it a go, this is how you can go about it.

Although there are many different scientific opinions on this, sixty-six days seems to be quite popular as the time required to acquire a new habit. This is just a bit more than two months.

Develop a walking plan

To acquire the walking habit you are going to need a plan, otherwise all the other priorities in your life will defeat your best intentions.

Your first step is to work out when you can fit in these walks. Although daily is ideal, even three to four times a week would be a good start.

To find the time to walk, you may need to be prepared to multitask. I sometimes make calls while I am walking to catch up with friends or attend to the odd business call. Zoom calls can work too.

I also arrange to walk with other people to catch up or discuss some business idea or proposition. So many business meetings these days are carried out over coffee in cafés. Why not walk and talk and then finish off with coffees?

Walking also can double as a creative time. You can record your thoughts and ideas on your phone to refer to later. I sometimes come up with some good writing ideas while out walking.

Instead of taking your car, if you have a destination within walking distance, walk it. Or if it is too far, drive half the way and walk the rest.

If you can establish a regular pattern of walking over a couple of months, it would be a good bet that you'd be hooked. If you are anything like me, you'd get cranky if you missed your daily walk.

Enough said; why not give it a go?

OTHER SPORTS AND PASTIMES

The following is a review of some of the most popular options.

Jogging – Walking's twin. While walking has low impact on your feet, legs and hips, jogging by comparison has high impact on these same areas. *Make sure that you wear good-quality track shoes recommended for your particular terrain. Get a specialist store to set you up.*

If you are a regular jogger or harrier, you will have superior cardiovascular capacity, agility and balance. Although you are likely to have strong legs, you may still be missing out in the areas of overall strength and flexibility.

Racquet sports – Tennis, badminton, squash and other racquet sports, because of their dynamic movements, have quite a high impact on your feet, legs and hips. This can cause issues in later life if these sports are played to excess.

They certainly give your body a great workout, including some of your core structures, and satisfy all of the BAFFS apart from flexibility.

Regular stretching to maintain or improve flexibility is essential if you play racquet sports regularly.

Swimming – A brilliant low-impact activity which also satisfies all of the BAFFS apart from overall flexibility. Water aerobics is in the same category and can include some stretches.

Contact sports – Rugby, football, basketball and other contact sports are fantastic for giving all of the BAFFS a great workout. Always include a good stretching routine before each practice or match.

Of course, these sports come with the dangers of a variety of injuries, with some of them, such as head injuries, impacting on players' future well-being.

While I love my rugby, I am well aware of the now well-documented brain damage that can result from the frequent collisions and which can cause early-onset dementia and other issues.

The speed and physicality of today's players exacerbates this risk, and we all hope that the rules and general management of the game can mitigate these risks as much as possible.

Snow sports and skate-boarding – What a fantastic range of options are now available, and the skills of some of the skiers, snowboarders, half-pipe exponents and others are awe-inspiring.

My advice for would-be exponents is to make sure you are competent in all of the BAFFS before heading on out there or up there.

Be it athletics or any other sport or pastime, by now you will have ascertained what area of BAFFS you might be missing out on with any particular activity.

VIC'S STORY

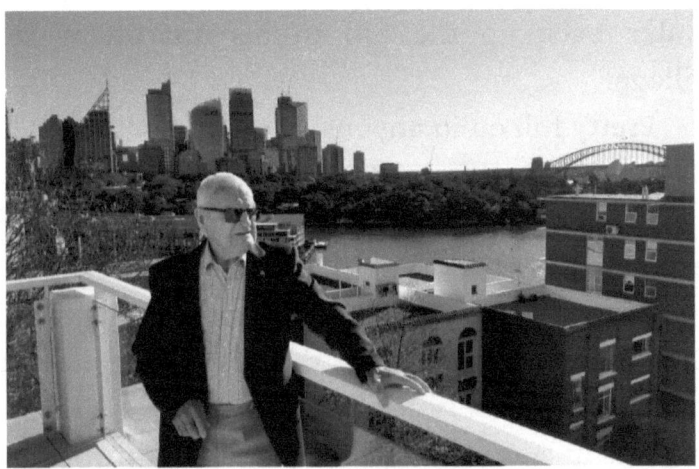

> I saw Vic one day at the ferry building in Devonport village waiting for the next ferry to Auckland city. He told me that he was off to Newmarket, which was a bus ride away from the Auckland ferry terminal.
>
> A couple of days later a friend of mine told me what Vic had been up to that day. He had gone to Newmarket to pick up some fish heads from the local fish shop there. This was with the view to burying

them in his garden plot allotment at the local organic gardens. Best fertiliser going, he reckoned.

So think about this. A three-kilometre walk to the ferry, fifteen minutes on the ferry, across the road to Britomart Station, a thirty-minute bus ride to Newmarket and a walk to the fish shop.

Vic picks up the fish heads and repeats his journey back to our village with the last kilometre being uphill.

He cuts up the fish heads and walks another kilometre down to his garden to bury them, then he walks back up the hill to his apartment at our village.

Pretty full on in anyone's book, I'd say, but all in a day's work for our ninety-six-year-old Vic. And just so typical of this tenacious fellow, who will always go the extra mile.

Born in 1938, Vic was brought up by his grandma. Like many youngsters in the war years, he started work aged just thirteen, in Auckland in 1942. His first job was in a Newmarket hardware store owned by the then mayor of Newmarket, Fred Philpott. Fred nearly had a heart attack one day when he spotted young Vic in a rather perilous position outside.

Tasked with cleaning the large front plate-glass window, Vic had positioned the top of the ladder slap in the middle of the glass. Fred appeared at the bottom of the ladder and told Vic to quietly make his way down.

After a couple of years, in 1947 Vic moved onto Diamond Retreads where he stayed for ten years.

Retreads were a great business to be in as new tyres were hard to come by.

Vic became engaged to his sweetheart Val in 1951 and they were married in 1953. They had managed to buy a section and used to go around looking at houses. If they saw one that they liked they would knock on the door and ask if they could have a look around. This practical approach paid off and they soon had their first home plans drawn up.

Most tenaciously, they spent the next few months making concrete blocks with just one mould. Vic said it was easy. Dry mix, tip it into the mould and then tip it out on a flat surface, just like you do with a sandcastle.

I googled the number of blocks needed for a two-bedroom house and the answer was two thousand plus!

The couple lived in a caravan on site while the house was being built. Vic and his father-in-law built the house together.

In 1957, Vic and Val rented out their house and moved to Tauranga in the Bay of Plenty. Their first child, Russell, was born in 1958. Soon after this, Val became homesick and they took the unique step of putting both their houses on the market. This was with the idea that whichever one sold first they would move into the other. With Val wanting to move back to Auckland, there appeared to be a bit of a flaw in this plan of theirs.

As luck would have it, the Tauranga house sold

first. They moved back to Auckland with six-week-old Russell.

Over the next thirty years the couple shifted around the country as Vic gathered great experience by working in various industries and positions.

He was never one to miss an opportunity. Vic saw an ad for Wattie's drivers in Auckland city. Disappointingly, on getting there he was told that the two drivers' positions had been given to two General Foods drivers. On finding out what branch, Vic immediately high-tailed it over to Epsom, and he was working as one of General Foods drivers the very next day.

Showing great versatility as he had never sold anything in his life, at General Foods he and a mate of his, Frank, shared the top billing in company sales each month.

Vic was transferred to Tauranga Tip Top and later onto Whakatāne; their daughter Vicky was born in November 1960. His journey continued with the same company when he was transferred to Nelson in 1967.

Vic and Val also had forays into business and in tourist town Rotorua they owned a lunch bar. It was a real family affair, and daughter Vicky, who was only eight at the time, could butter bread faster than any of the staff. Obviously talented then, she has gone on to become the principal of a large secondary school on the North Shore of Auckland.

Always on the lookout for a good business, Vic spotted an opportunity while driving for Tip Top. He noted that the store at Fox Glacier had sold 8000 postcards between Christmas and March that year. Sadly, someone bought the store before Vic could make an offer.

Shortly after this they moved back to Tauranga and bought the Matua Dairy, which they ran for a number of years.

Vic could turn his hand to virtually anything. Among other things, he managed a branch of a frozen foods company, owned a taxi, and was a volunteer fireman and ambulance driver.

At age fifty-nine Vic suffered his first minor heart attack, and this slowed him down a bit. Living in the North Island country town of Ngatea, he drove school buses part time and packed kiwifruit in the local packhouse.

If there is anything that requires infinite patience and a wide range of skills, it is the business of restoring vintage cars. Vic lovingly restored a 1924 Morris Cowley and a 1926 Chrysler.

Another heart attack and a life-threatening aneurysm in 2010 saw Vic and Val move back to Auckland to help Vicky with her family. Vic was retired by then, and Vicky and her husband Quentin bought an apartment for them in Auckland. Val passed away in 2018. They were three months off being married for sixty-five years.

Some of Vic's reflections on his life include a feeling that he would have achieved more in life if he had had a better education. Well, although that may have been the case, I think anyone would agree that he has had a spectacular life so far and achieved many different things in many ways.

Around our village there are numerous opportunities for social activities. Vic is a mainstay of many of them and can be found at our own watering hole, Billy's Bar, most days that it is open.

He played league as a young man and bowls for thirty years and told me that he would like to play more sport or even help out at a business that needed help.

Sounds like Vic, contemplating coming out of retirement in his nineties. Well, why not?

Ryman Villages across Australasia recently held a walking challenge whereby you had to record your local walks to total the sixty-kilometre length of the Abel Tasman Coast Track in thirty-one days. The Abel Tasman National Park encompasses a beautiful coastal walk in the north-west of the South Island.

You guessed it. Vic was right into this and completed the journey in eleven days. This placed him in the top hundred out of many hundreds of competitors.

A group of us walked with Vic on his last day to celebrate his achievement. He proudly told us that his best day was over eight kilometres. Bear in mind also that Devonport is a fairly hilly little suburb.

I visit Vic in his apartment to do an audio recording of his life. I notice many colourful spools of wool piled up in an armchair and a couple of equally colourful wool rugs on the floor. Just using a small tool, he hand-makes the rugs and gives them away to family and friends. He has been doing this for thirty years and also makes them to be raffled for charity. The last beneficiary was for prostate cancer.

Vic is a kind-hearted, quiet achiever who has positively touched many people during his long lifetime. And what a great attitude and zest for life he has, and no doubt there are plenty more adventures in store for this terrific nonagenarian.

7
BUILDING RESILIENCE

KEY POINTS

- In my reckoning, the more resilient you are, the more likely you are to be able to get the best out of the rest of your life.
- The people whose stories I have featured all demonstrate a resilience and zest for life. They also exhibit being a healthy weight, fit, getting regular exercise, and having a purpose in life and a positive attitude. And they are all well connected to friends and family on a daily basis.
- Like brushing your teeth every day, resilient people will do some form of physical activity most days of their lives. I think that this is a key factor in extending your healthspan as far as possible.
- I am convinced that resilient people will inevitably cope

better with life's challenges and lead happier and healthier lives.

BOUNCING BACK

The definition of resilience is your ability to cope with and bounce back from life's challenges.

If you are a very resilient person, you will still experience all the physical and psychological fears that a less resilient person will feel. You will just be better prepared to deal with them and bounce back more quickly.

In essence, all of the chapters so far in this book have been designed to help you to build resilience. The rest of this chapter aims to drill down into all of the key aspects of this crucial concept.

Considering that our complex lives in today's world can be full of difficulties, your ability to be resilient will play a massive part in your life. And it can mean the difference between having a happy, well-connected and contented life to the absolute opposite.

While resilience can be an innate genetic quality, it also involves the learning of skills. If you already have a high level of resilience, you are sure to recognise these traits as you read on. And you might just learn one or two new skills.

Life's problems can come in many forms and cause various levels of physical and mental anguish. Thankfully, successfully coping with any of these crises means that you will employ the same set of skills time after time.

Sounds easy, doesn't it? But not so fast. Ideally, you will first need to have reasonable levels of competence in some key areas. I'm really talking about some of the topics that we have already covered in this book.

These are the basic building blocks to put you into a good position to be able to cope with what life throws at you. Building up your resilience skills will just add that layer of completion at the top.

If, for example, you still suffer from denial of death, have feelings of immortality, are in poor physical condition and still drink like a fish and eat heaps of junk food, you may need to rethink your life first.

TEN TRAITS OF RESILIENT PEOPLE

These are not in any particular order of importance. Many of these have already been covered earlier in the book, particularly in the chapter on attitude.

1. Connection

You will be well connected and value and care about the relationships you have with friends and family.

You are also likely to be an active social media user to enable regular contact with loved ones who you live away from.

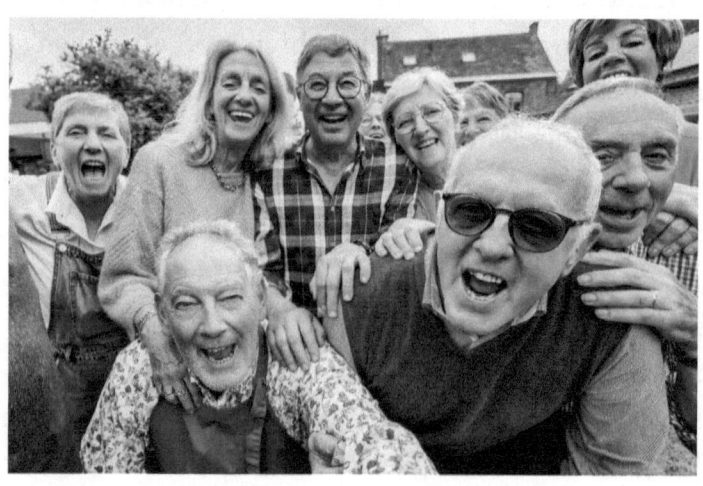

We have already talked about the Grant Study in our chapter on attitude. This has been running for eighty years and examines the lives of hundreds of male Harvard graduates and a large group of more underprivileged men. It overwhelmingly proves that strong and loving relationships across the board are far and away the most important factor in people's health, happiness and longevity.

It also says rather starkly that 'loneliness kills'.

I personally have never felt really lonely and have a great deal of sympathy for those who do. Adding to this loneliness can be apprehensive feelings about meeting with strangers in different situations.

One really good way of overcoming this is to either join a club which involves something you are interested in, like a sport or a cultural activity. You are still with strangers; the difference now is that you immediately have something in common with them.

The same would apply if you were volunteering at say an op shop or other community charitable organisation. You are all there for the same reason and with one united goal in mind.

Closer to home in your own neighbourhood, if you do not know the people in your street perhaps talk to a few and there may be interest in having a street party or something similar.

Through the various media outlets, we know a lot about wars and other international news from far-flung places without even knowing our next-door neighbour!

2. Positive attitude

You are optimistic and positive most of the time and have a great attitude to life. We have already covered this in some detail in our attitude chapter. This sort of attitude is a real asset when things get tough, and you are likely to be quite a naturally resilient type.

If you are a negative and pessimistic type of person, it will be more difficult to bounce back when problems arise. The key here is your recognition of this bent. Once you are aware that your attitude will not help you to recover from a tricky situation, the more likely you are to be able to find a solution.

3. Fitness

You will place considerable importance on being physically fit and are likely to be quite proficient in each of the five BAFFS. This is a real asset when the going gets tough.

4. Living in the present

You mostly live in the present and focus and are present in your day-to-day relationships with friends. It is unhealthy to dwell too often on the past, particularly if this involves negative stuff like stressing out over missed opportunities.

You can certainly learn from experiences, both good and bad. Resilient people will use the past positively and learn from past difficulties and enjoy the fond memories with family and friends.

If you live in the present, you are seeing clearly that moment in real time. Whatever the context, whether it is maybe the brilliance of a sporting moment, a colourful bird flying by or anything else, you are in there living it first-hand.

If you are being continually distracted by other things that are happening in your life, you will often miss out on life itself.

5. Good listening

Resilient people are very likely to be good listeners. When you are talking to them, they will be giving you their full and undivided attention. As we have just discussed, they are present. They might not always agree with what you have to say, and they may find what you have to say quite boring.

People who are poor listeners miss out on so much. They are often distracted by other things that are going on in their mind or around them. I think the biggest sin of all is not really listening but more biding time until it is your turn.

Often these people are only looking to push their own agenda, and this is quite insulting to the person who is talking to them. And it is oh so obvious and tiresome.

Resilient people are curious and interested in what other people have to say. This is a wonderful asset in helping to build strong connections with other people.

I don't think anyone could claim to be the perfect listener all of the time. We all have times where we are distracted by other things going on in our minds and not fully cognisant of what's being said. But a good listener will be someone who most times will be present and listening carefully. A poor listener is someone who most times is distracted and most times is only looking to tell their side of the story.

6. Flexibility

You are flexible, know your limits and able to make other plans.

You may have set your heart on something and worked hard to achieve it. It will not always come to pass. Sometimes you miss out. It is important that you have the ability to accept this, maybe learn some lessons from it, and move on.

You will have read the story of the famous athletics coach Arch Jelley earlier, and he talked with me about 'using the difficulty'.

Arch let his driver's licence lapse when he turned 100. Only a short time later his wife Rachel lost her licence and so 'they were without wheels'. They used this difficulty by walking more and getting fitter and actually saving money.

In my case recently, being diagnosed with a back condition meant that continuing to play golf and tennis could mean further deterioration. Knowing my limits and unwilling to take this risk, I gave up both. After a lifetime of playing these sports, this was pretty tough. I used the difficulty by undertaking various exercises and stretches to strengthen my back.

At the same time, I started to put far more time into golf croquet and have the opportunity to become a much better player in what is a relatively new sport for me.

After six months of core strengthening rehab and getting the nod from my back specialist, I am delighted to be back playing golf, albeit with a much-abbreviated swing.

Having just recently been reminded by Arch about the possibilities of turning a difficult situation to his advantage helped me to do the same. There are so many aspects of your life where negative stuff pops up. Rather than reluctantly accepting your fate, if you have the ability to turn these to your advantage the difference is quite massive.

Evidently Covid gave many people the opportunity to take time to re-evaluate their careers with many deciding to completely change direction. They used the difficulty which Covid presented and moved from careers they were unhappy with to a new field.

Being open and flexible means that you will always be better equipped to deal with life's inevitable disappointments and crises.

7. Self-reliance

You like spending time on your own. This sounds counter-intuitive to the other resilience measure of being well connected. What it means is that in our busy, complex and connected lives, time on our own can be a wonderful change. On the other hand, a person who craves others' attention and company at all times may have some self-worth issues.

This can be the one-on-one situation of co-dependency. This is where time away from each other causes problems like feeling a lack of self-worth. Or it can be in the wider context of one person almost fearing being left alone away from their normal network of work colleagues, friends and family.

In both cases this is a real shame, because time away from the day-to-day hurly-burly of workplaces and homes can be a precious and sometimes well-earned commodity.

If you feel that you may have become co-dependent, it may be worth talking to your partner or those close to you as to how they view this and, if necessary, seek some counselling.

On the other hand, resilient people will jump at the chance to spend some quality time on their own and have no qualms about it.

8. Ability to say no

You are able to say no. Oh my gosh, it can be so difficult when someone close to you puts you on the spot and you just do not like to say no. Even though you know that you probably should.

I remember well a few years ago coaching a high-ranking executive in the health sector. Call him John. After doing the usual fact finding, I could see that John was seriously stressed out by his workload, constantly having to bring work home and stretching out precious time with his wife very thinly. This was causing ongoing issues with what had formerly been a close and loving relationship.

What coaching is all about is to get the solutions from your client by asking the right open-ended questions. It can be as simple as saying, 'What do you think the biggest problem here is?'

After a bit of thought, John said something like, 'Well, I think I am the biggest problem.' And so it turned out to be. Even though he was the boss, he was taking on far more responsibility than he needed to.

Most of this turned out to be his inability to say no. He worked out a simple strategy for himself. If approached by someone to do something, if he was unsure at all about doing this, he would say something like, 'I'll have to think about this, and will come back to you.'

This allowed him the time to think it through before coming back to that person or group. John found that by doing this he ended up delegating some of these requests to his own staff. In other cases, after thinking it through he would accept if it was appropriate.

He was pleasantly surprised at how his workload seemed to diminish, he stopped taking work home at nights and he and his wife enjoyed far more free time together.

Breaking this cycle was as simple as that. Little things can make a big difference. If you are someone like John, who often says yes when you should be saying no, just try this. It works.

9. Gratitude

You are grateful for what you have. This concept has popped up a couple of times earlier in the book. You can easily get sucked into the world of negativity that surrounds us with the seemingly endless media coverage of wars, storms, fires, politics and much more.

I get sucked into this too and need to make a conscious effort to focus on what the positive elements of my life really are. And as you get older and have to give up stuff, focus on what you can do, not what you can no longer do.

I have a list of things in my head that I am truly grateful for and when things get a bit bumpy, cheer myself up by thinking about these truly positive things in my life.

10. You have purpose in your life

We have already covered this topic in our earlier chapter on attitude. I have gained some fascinating insights from reading about Okinawan women who pursue their ikigai. I hope you do too.

Okinawa is one of the islands of Japan and ikigai – finding

meaning and purpose – is practised widely across the island by their women who amazingly have an average life expectancy of ninety years.

One of the primary elements of traditional Japanese medicine is that your physical well-being is directly affected by mental and emotional health. A state of well-being can be achieved by the devotion and mastery of activities that you enjoy and that also bring a sense of achievement. So ikigai is a reason to get up in the morning!

If you practise ikigai well, you are likely to experience a sense of having worth and gaining benefits by taking part in these activities that you already enjoy.

In a sporting sense, you hear sportspeople talk about being 'in the zone'. They have a brilliant feeling of flow and are able to effortlessly perform a string of best moments one after the other.

No matter what your own level of sport is or has been, you will understand and clearly remember your own highlights. And that's what it can be. Your own amazing highlights reel.

In golf it was that time you broke ninety for the first time and effortlessly drained long putts all over the course.

That time you made that snooker break of twenty-four and potted nine consecutive balls. Normally you'd struggle to pot three in a row. And better still was the look on the face of your mate when you beat him for the first time.

Or that time your cellar-dweller netball team effortlessly beat the competition's leading team, and you scored the winning goal with a long-range shot.

The Okinawan women's range of activities which they love and are good at would be wide and varied and no doubt encompass cultural, sporting and many other fields.

An added benefit occurs when the activity brings value to others. A further less altruistic benefit occurs when you actually get paid for it.

How to practise ikigai

You first write down activities that you really like and are good at – or even potentially good at with a bit of practice.

Work out a plan of how you can regularly take part in these activities and improve your performance. And better still if they help other people and even better if you can get paid for doing it.

If you are still working and really enjoy your occupation, this is a great benefit. If you are still working and do not enjoy your work, the ikigai principles would mean that you could spend some time looking at more pleasurable options.

Reviewing my own situation, I worked out that I really enjoy writing and seem to be quite good at it. This book has been a brilliant project and could potentially help a lot of people. If you are one of these and are reading these words today after buying the book, well, I have achieved the other ikigai benefit – I am getting paid for my efforts.

SHERILYN'S STORY

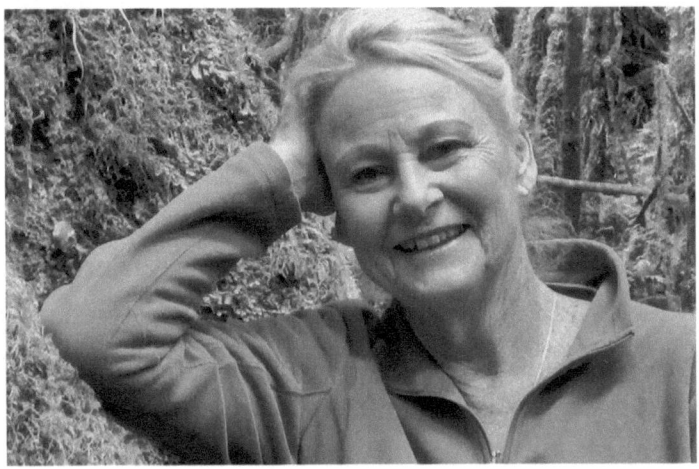

> I first met Sherilyn in 2021 when she moved into our retirement village. I soon discovered that she was quite the force of nature.
>
> We have both agreed that building resilience is one of the cornerstones of having a happy and healthy life. Her story is a fitting one to back-end this chapter and contains many examples of what resilience is all about.
>
> At the local croquet club, she was soon volunteering to knock their gardens into shape and much weeding, trimming and planting followed. She doubles as a waitress at the croquet club social fund-raising evenings too. Also, she and a small group of residents have ensured that our recycling room is now brilliantly ordered, and woe betide anyone who puts those pesky batteries or wine tops in the wrong containers.

After a lifetime of treating many bodies as a neuro-physiotherapist, she admits that she still observes unsuspecting residents who could benefit from some form of therapy.

Her father was in the police overseas, and her mother worked in various clinics to support women and children's welfare.

After the war, her parents were stationed in the state of Sabah in northern Borneo for twenty years. Advised that their first child should be born in England, Sherilyn was born in London in 1952. Her brother John was born in Sabah, eighteen months later.

She had an amazing childhood with lots of adventures and, at times, a fair amount of responsibility heaped upon her young shoulders.

In Sabah she and John were first home-schooled then went to primary school followed by boarding school in England, at age nine.

In Sabah, they had wonderful times picnicking and playing around the beautiful white-sand beaches, searching the reefs for cowrie shells, swimming in the rivers, and riding friends' ponies.

When their parents had leave from Sabah, once every three years the family would spend time in the New Forest in Hampshire.

'These times were magical with no devices and where imagination was your friend. We had so much freedom and would bike for miles with our friends and have adventures in the forest.

'Brother John was a daredevil and had many near scrapes. One winter he very nearly drowned. We were riding near a quarry and, typically, John decided to tear off down the very steep quarry slope and bike across the ice. To our horror, halfway across, the ice broke and he and his bike disappeared into the freezing water. Somehow, we got him out, although the bike was never recovered.

'Our third holiday of the year was spent in "holiday homes" for children whose parents were overseas. There was not much love going around and felt almost Dickensian.'

If they did not eat their fruit and vegetables, they would have to remain at the table until they did. Sherilyn used to bring an envelope with her and shovel the peas and apricots into it and hide it away.

I asked her whether she eats her fruit and vegetables now. She admitted that this all changed when she had children of her own and they had asked her the same question.

From age nine Sherilyn and John would fly between Sabah and England to attend boarding school twice a year.

'These flights caused me a lot of anxiety and I felt very responsible for my younger brother. There was not much in the way of guidance from the airline staff.

On the plane, we ate virtually nothing as we didn't like the food and would pretend to be asleep when meals were brought around. We would be disturbed by a hostess saying, "Your mother says you must at least have a glass of milk."'

On occasion they would stay overnight in a hotel and many hours were spent in airports. You can only imagine how frightening this must have been for these youngsters in those large echoing spaces with people rushing hither and thither.

Sherilyn remained in boarding school until she was seventeen. After her parents had returned to England, she spent her sixth-form year in Hampshire, as a day pupil at a co-ed school.

'I remember at boarding school earlier on spending time trying to cheer up homesick children who used to cry at night. So this caring gene was apparent in my DNA even way back then.'

Sherilyn's father had mentioned that she might make a good physio. She had no idea why and she took him up on it, and an excellent idea it turned out to be.

During her first year at physiotherapy school in London, she boarded at the YMCA. After this she went flatting with some physio friends and remembers the freezing flat and their combined lack of cooking skills which led to much cheese on toast.

After three years at a rehab hospital in Wiltshire, she moved to New Zealand and took a position at Sunnyside Psychiatric Hospital in Christchurch.

'It was a matter of learning on the job as I had no experience in this field. I had to learn a very unique set of skills quickly, to deal with the effects of mental dysfunction, with the care and kindness required to gain their trust.

'I was very immature and naïve at the time and things could get a bit tricky. I was thrust in front of an exercise class of perhaps twenty patients, and had to take it in my stride when approached with the comment, "Who do you think you are telling me what to do?" I could have answered that I had no idea as I had been given no guidelines as to what to do.

'I remember another chap coming up to me and saying, "You can captain my ship anytime!"

'Most of the patients had poor coordination and really no awareness of where their body began and ended. I had them draw a stick figure in their assessment and compared this with a stick figure drawn at the end of six weeks of exercises. The second stick figure was much more realistic.

'My daughter was born in Christchurch in 1979 and my son Robert in Southampton, UK twenty months later. We moved back to New Zealand in 1981 when Robert was ten weeks old.

'I had a part-time job at a private hospital and in a private respiratory practice before approaching Middlemore Hospital looking for a job, where they welcomed me with open arms – no formal interview, just told to go and get measured for a uniform.'

After fourteen years in the Rehabilitation Unit in Middlemore, Sherilyn moved to Mangawhai and took up a senior position at Whangarei Base Hospital in their rehab ward. By this time the children had left home and she was divorced from her husband.

In 2009 her second husband, Michael, was diagnosed with Hodgkin's lymphoma and Sherilyn stopped work in 2014 to care for him full time. Michael passed away in 2016 and she moved to Devonport in Auckland in 2021 to William Sanders Village to be closer to both her children who lived in Auckland.

The second half of Sherilyn's story is about her quite brilliant career as a physio. Typically, she will tell me off for the word 'brilliant' but perhaps you will judge for yourself.

I had shown her my chapter on 'resilience' and we had both agreed that it was a key factor in anyone's recovery from illness or injury. This becomes a common theme as we take a look back at her career. We will start off with some more memorable patient success stories.

'I remember a double amputee giving me a big hug of thanks many years later in the local dairy. I was thrilled to hear that he was successfully mobile and living alone. People don't realise the incredible amount of energy it takes to walk with prosthetics. I also received a hug at my local supermarket from another amputee, years after his rehab.'

Receiving heartfelt feedback from stroke patients in the community as they recalled their early physio rehab was also rewarding.

'I have kept a beautifully written letter of gratitude from an ex-prisoner whose rehab journey was a real challenge. He hated the British, which was not a good start, and was hell bent on making a bomb to blow us all up. Women didn't rate that highly either and at that stage he was an undiagnosed schizophrenic.

'On a home visit, it was discovered he was growing a crop of marijuana in a spare room.

He wanted to know the Latin names of the muscles we focused on which was a bit unusual, and he became highly motivated in his rehab.

I had another stroke patient who had severe impairments and could only say the words 'Jesus Christ'. I learnt to understand what he meant by the inflection he put on these words. He visited the hospital some months later and, while I was working with another patient, I heard in the corridor the cry "Jesus Christ" and knew immediately he was meaning "Where is she?" What a joyful hug that was.'

The patients in these success stories certainly were grateful for their excellent treatment, positive about their lives and had obviously grown to know their own limits. All of these are key factors in resilience and without these their outcomes would certainly have been less positive.

Then of course there were the inevitable disappointments and dilemmas.

'I vividly remember a 28-year-old double amputee on dialysis, nearly blind, little strength in his arms or legs, or sensation in his hands. He was an angry young Māori man who had not heeded any of the early-warning signs clearly signalled by his doctors.

'He had been quite rightly told by the prosthetists at the Auckland Limb Centre that he would never walk efficiently again, as it would just be too demanding on his failing body. The necessary effort to walk, by a "high" double amputee, requires roughly two hundred percent more energy than that of a non-amputee.

'He certainly knew his rights and his aggressive personality proved to be a huge challenge for everyone as he demanded a new set of legs.

'With enormous perseverance from us both he could walk a short distance on a heavy-duty customised gutter frame. I'll never forget the look on the faces of the nurses in the dialysis unit when he walked through their doors. With "legs", at six-foot four, he was quite a different proposition to the man that they were used to seeing wheeled through the door in a wheelchair.

'As bloody minded as he was, once he got home he never walked again because it was easier and quicker to get around in a wheelchair.

'This case was also memorable as it brought up for me the dilemma of beneficence, which is the obligation to act for the benefit of the patient and to support a number of moral rules to protect and defend the rights of others.

'His cost to the hospital would have been in the hundreds of thousands of dollars for, in the end, not a lot of benefit to the patient!

'On the resilience scale he scored poorly as his body condition was irretrievable in a functional sense.

'While most amputees were compliant, some of the smokers certainly weren't. They would often go out for a smoke during their rehab stay, even after being warned that continuing to smoke would likely mean they would lose their other leg in two to five years. And sure enough, they would return some years later to have the other leg off. This sure is a tough addiction to conquer.

'Sometimes having great resilience is just not enough. A young, fit man with everything going for him was admitted, diagnosed with a rare genetic condition which caused him to suffer repeated strokes. Although he never spoke again, rehab had him back on his feet and walking. Continued strokes meant further deterioration, sadly, and a revision of goals. This highly resilient man died in his fifties. He was concerned the disease may have been passed on to his daughters.

'During the eighties while I was working at Middlemore a Tongan gentleman was flown to New Zealand for rehab. I worked with him for six weeks. It was a great pleasure as I had lived in Tonga as a teenager, while my father worked with the police force there. It was like treating family and he finally returned to Tonga walking with a stick.

'As a "rehab novice" I had forgotten to consider the relevance of his being the head of a Tongan family. He was waited on hand and foot by his family and lost a lot of his independence and probably physical abilities. If they had been present during his rehab, we would have established relevant goals, perhaps.

'There is no doubt in my mind that a key factor in how well a patient recovers depends on how resilient they are. It's having the mental fortitude to cope with the trauma and hardship and find meaning to this altered life to which you have to adapt. It requires optimism, determination and improved self-awareness to conquer the new challenges that you have to confront.

'I wonder, too, how much resilience is genetic and how much is learnt, and also the importance of social connection. Content in my own company, I have to push myself to get out and about and socialise in different situations.

'When I learned about your BAFFS concept for improving physical functionality it was an ah-ha moment. "Practise what you preach!" It gave me the impetus to work out the areas I was weak in and look to improve in these.

'I'm really enjoying my aquarobics and two yoga sessions a week, which I had never considered before, and I continue to walk at least five kilometres as often as possible. This will improve my fitness, flexibility, balance and strength and lift my spirits, with a view to a healthier life.'

As you have seen, Sherilyn's career was wide ranging and also included the setting up of the Northland Amputee Service and contributing to the standards of a new acute stroke ward. She was also involved in teaching the principles of care for stroke and amputee rehabilitation to physio, nursing and medical students and other healthcare professionals.

Some of Sherilyn's views on how you should treat patients are as follows.

'As the saying goes, "If at first you don't succeed then try, try, try again." I used to say to my students that it may not be just the patient who has plateaued but maybe the therapist too. Try harder to find ways that will lead to success.

'Being mindful of cultural issues, and continued encouragement and humour are vitally important. I felt chameleon-like, adapting my style to suit different personalities. Straight talking to the bolshie, relaxing words to the timid and anxious, and always kind, respectful and professional. Give 100 per cent to them every time, no matter how you feel.'

Sherilyn certainly has had a colourful and varied life, living in different countries, and touching so many people so positively wherever she went.

And if you ever have the pleasure of meeting her, if you are feeling at all under the weather, a little limp or a grimace will almost certainly result in you receiving some first-class care.

What a real privilege and a pleasure to be able to write Sherilyn's story!

Thinking about resilience has led me to recall some of the conversations and experiences I have had with Arch, who is a centenarian, and June, Vic, Margaret, Pat and other nonagenarians who have generously added their life stories to my book.

I have noticed several elements which all of these people have in common. Although fairly ancient in human terms, they all still have a real vibrancy and zest for life. It seems to sort of shine out of them.

I recall a photo Margaret sent me of her at her local golf club, proudly posing with her shiny new driver that was almost as tall as her. Grinning cheekily, standing straight as a die and quite pert in her black beret, checked trousers and matching white jacket and golf shoes.

I rang her to compliment her on the photo and asked how she had played. 'Did you walk?' I asked, knowing full well what she would say.

'Is there any other way?' was her answer, which kind of says it all.

I think of June at age ninety-eight, having recently recovered from a serious bout of influenza, walking serenely down the corridor with her colourful cane. Hair beautifully coiffed and stylishly dressed in a chic pink dress with matching shoes.

She orders a red wine at the bar and joins her two equally well-turned-out old friends to make a trio we call the three dames. Getting togged up like this requires some effort and June just manages this day in day out. It's quite inspiring and fantastic really.

Another key aspect I have observed is that of the regularity of their exercise. Without fail, Arch does 100 squats and walks every day. June swims every day, Margaret either golfs, walks or gardens most days of the week. Vic walks to his garden and back most days.

Part Two
PHYSICAL AND BIOLOGICAL MATTERS

1
PHYSICAL FUNCTIONALITY

KEY POINTS

- This chapter provides a brief on what to look for as far as your physical functionality is concerned. It will help you to rate where you are up to and highlight any areas of concern, providing a physical 'warrant of fitness'.
- BAFFS is a convenient acronym for all aspects of your physical being. They are balance, agility, fitness (cardiovascular), flexibility and strength.
- Your very independence relies on you having sufficient balance to avoid falls, agility to sidestep imminent disasters, enough cardiovascular puff to climb up stairs, good flexibility and sufficient strength to cope with your day-to-day physical needs.
- When you are young you set yourself up with a huge bank of physical skills and resources. These are easily

retained through all of your school years as you refine your choices of games and sports and other physical activities.

- When you reach adulthood, life seems to get in the road of everything. Cracks may start to appear. It's worth remembering that we all naturally begin to incrementally go downhill from age thirty.
- This decline can be dramatically slowed by regular attention to your BAFFS, for instance. The trick is to be mindful of this and pay attention to the everyday clues that you are getting which signal that all is not well.
- De-training – This means reduced physical activity from what you are used to. You will lose muscle strength and size, your blood pressure can increase, your cardiovascular fitness reduces and other medical markers can be affected.
- Illness or injury – Many people may compromise or sometimes permanently lose those functions even when they recover.
- Do not give away any aspect of your BAFFS without a fight.
- Working your way back to where you were helps to build resilience and retains those crucial physical functionality levels.
- A constant reality check on what's really going on here is essential. And make sure that you act on your findings.

PHYSICAL FUNCTIONALITY (PF) AND BAFFS

This chapter will provide a brief on what to look for as far as your own physical functionality is concerned. It will help you to rate where you are up to and highlight any areas that may be of concern. It will provide a physical 'warrant of fitness' if you like. **BAFFS** is a convenient acronym for all aspects of your physical being: balance, agility, fitness (cardiovascular), flexibility and strength. Collectively these are at the heart of your PF, especially as you grow older.

Your very independence relies on you having sufficient balance to avoid falls, agility to sidestep imminent disasters, enough cardiovascular puff to climb up stairs, good flexibility and sufficient strength to cope with your day-to-day physical needs.

Let's take a closer look at some examples of what happens in our lives.

We will start off with a newborn child. Dad has done his bit and with Mum doing the heavy lifting, the miracle of life occurs.

Baby starts on the floor and learns the basic manoeuvring skills of turning over, and crawling. And then 'ta-da', the landmark moment: baby up on its feet and creating an instant social-media storm.

From there it's a steep learning curve with many milestones. Trees to climb, bikes and skateboards to ride, learning to swim, sport to play – it's all great fun.

As a growing child, you are setting yourself up with a huge bank of physical skills and resources. They are easily retained through all of your school years as you refine your choices of games, sports and other physical activities.

Of course, in our modern world of screens and games consoles, this physically active life can be stifled or cut short by countless hours on these machines. This is a great pity, and these countless hours of sitting are a worrying sign for the physical future of these sedentary-before-their-time types.

LIFE GETS IN THE WAY

Adulthood beckons. All too soon school days are over. You are either off to travel the world, begin your working life or going to university or other tertiary institution.

Soon life seems to get in the road of everything. You start accumulating assets, like a car, a pension fund and mortgages. Hand in hand come insurances, rates and a whole host of other pesky responsibilities that seem to occupy your every waking moment.

Although I have over-egged that last paragraph a bit, and most people cope quite admirably, you will certainly know what I mean.

And being married with children creates a whole new exciting and complex set of challenges.

Life gets in the way of everything and there just seems to be so many competing priorities.

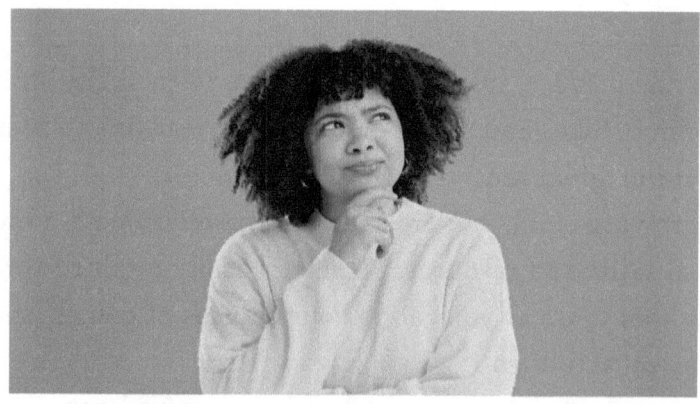

Cracks can start to appear, and it's worth remembering that we all naturally begin to go incrementally downhill from age thirty.

We also know that that this decline can be dramatically slowed down by regular attention to your BAFFS, for instance. The trick is to be mindful of this and pay attention to the everyday clues that you are getting which signal that all is not well. In your busy complex world, it is easier to gloss over these physical imperfections and in this case, ignorance will not end up in bliss.

Unknowingly, you will start to compromise in some areas of physicality and posture.

As a kid you are always playing and pushing the boundaries of physicality. Climbing trees, skateboarding, play fighting, running, and many other pursuits mean you are building, training, exercising and testing your full range of physical attributes.

Eventually, however, all of your wide-ranging physicality takes a back seat, and your adult life takes over. Having said this, there are still plenty of exceptions to this generalisation in the form of athletes and dedicated sportspeople.

I believe the overwhelming majority will fall into the other category. You will know where you fit in. If you were a normal active kid, you will still have an excellent bank of physical attributes which for a while will stand you in good stead.

FIGHT BACK

De-training means reduced physical activity from what you are used to. It doesn't just apply to athletes. You will lose muscle strength and size, your blood pressure can increase, your cardiovascular fitness reduces, and other medical markers can be affected.

Illness or injury – As I write this, I am experiencing a painful bout of sciatica. It doesn't help that I am on a cruise ship in the middle of the Coral Sea.

Having to sit down while I dry my feet, and put socks or trousers on, is annoying but necessary because of the pain. Once I recover, I will be endeavouring to regain these lost bits of physical functionality as quickly as possible.

Many people during adversity in the form of illness or injuries will compromise like I'm doing, and sometimes permanently lose those functions even when they recover.

Do not give away any aspect of your BAFFS without a fight. Working your way back to where you were helps to build resilience and retains those crucial physical functionality levels.

Don't resign yourself to it. Don't say, 'Oh well, it's just so easy to sit on the bed and put my socks on.' Fight back and don't go quietly. If your best efforts fail, at least you've done your best.

REALITY CHECK

We have covered death denial earlier, something that can be a handicap when facing the realities of life. You conveniently shut out some of the signs that cracks are appearing and simply don't pay attention.

After all, you're kidding yourself that you are immortal. Bad things are just not happening.

A constant check on what's really going on here is essential. And make sure that you act on your findings.

Your reality checklist – The following is a list of normal human losses of physical function as we age. See how you are faring.

- Reaching back for your seat belt is becoming just a little difficult.
- You need to be careful getting in and out of your car as you are feeling a bit stiff.
- You are finding it tricky turning your head and shoulders to see out the back window. Thank heavens for that reversing camera.
- You find that you are letting your hand rest on the handrail now as you come down the stairs.
- You were a bit puffed going up those three flights of stairs the other day. In fact, you always take the lift now if you can. It's much easier.
- Some of your friends are now using a golf cart so you've joined them and no longer walk the course. It was starting to get difficult.
- You just can't seem to get the length off the tee that you used to.
- Instead of standing on one leg to put your sock on, you now sit on the bed.
- The same goes for putting on your pants.
- You've put a chair in the bathroom for the same reason as it is too difficult to dry your foot standing on one leg.
- You are now putting your hands on the edge of the bath so that you can get your legs over and into the bath.
- You notice that it is now difficult to get up off a low seat.
- At the beach last year, you had difficulty standing up after coming out of the water.
- And the same goes for standing up after sitting on the grass or a floor.

- Your feet seem to be further away now when you are clipping your toenails. In fact, it's quite a stretch to do this.
- You need to be careful to retain your balance when walking on uneven ground.
- You can't touch your toes with straight legs.
- In the garden you do your weeding by kneeling on a towel.
- You are a bit unsteady up the ladder cleaning out the gutters.
- An hour or two in the garden makes you feel tired and stiff.
- You were watching your granddaughter play hopscotch the other day and had a feeling that your days of hopping from one place to another might be over.

How did you get on? All still a piece of cake or are some of these day-to-day activities really becoming more difficult?

This is quite a good reality check. The good news is that, if a few cracks are appearing, it is relatively easy to put matters right.

2

THE PHYSICAL FOUNDATION BLOCKS

KEY POINTS

- Your body is made up of fat, lean tissue (muscles and organs), bones, and water.
- Lean tissue can be lost in your muscles, liver, kidney, and other organs. Bones often become less dense, and your amount of body fat often incrementally increases.
- From age thirty, you start to incrementally deteriorate in several areas. Gravity plays a significant part in all of this, and you can actually become shorter.
- Weaker leg muscles and stiffer joints can make moving around harder. Excess body fat and changes in body shape can also affect your balance.
- You can delay this incremental decay by paying attention to the key cornerstones of BAFFS: balance, agility, cardiovascular fitness, flexibility and strength.

- If you can preserve and maintain a good level of competence and fitness in these crucial areas, you will be giving yourself a better chance of having a much greater quality of life in your later years.
- This will help to increase your healthspan years and lower your biological age.
- A real bonus is that many activities will provide benefits for at least one or even all of the BAFFS. For example, all of your BAFFS will be catered for in a morning's gardening.
- A reasonable level of ability in all of the BAFFS is essential.

GRADUAL LOSS

Your body is made up of fat, lean tissue (muscles and organs), bones, and water.

From age thirty, you start to incrementally deteriorate in several areas. Lean tissue can be lost in muscles, liver, kidneys, and other organs. This loss is called atrophy. Bones often become less dense and the amount of body fat often incrementally increases. As you know, this added body fat seems to centre itself round your middle.

Muscle will burn energy (calories) at double the rate fat will. This loss of muscle mass and corresponding accumulation of fat is a double whammy, and it also causes your basal metabolic rate (BMR) to slow down. This also negatively affects your ability to burn calories. Your basal metabolic rate) is the minimum number of calories your body needs to maintain basic, life-sustaining functions while at complete rest. It is a measure of the rate at which all of your bodily processes operate.

Gravity plays a significant part in all of this, and many of your bits and bobs seem to gradually go south, and wrinkles and rolls become abundant.

With the double whammy of your loss of strength from ageing and the compressing of your vertebrae, you can become shorter. Some older people can become up to seven to eight centimetres shorter.

Weaker leg muscles and stiffer joints can make moving around harder. Excess body fat and changes in body shape can also affect your balance. These body changes can make falls more likely.

Even at the elite level of sportspeople, the fast twitches seem to gradually evaporate, with perhaps the odd exception being someone like Roger Federer. With contact sports like rugby and gridiron, it is even more noticeable as multiple injuries take their toll. Even the great All Black rugby first-five Dan Carter, at age thirty-eight, had noticeably slowed down from his former epic best.

On a good day, I used to be able to hit a golf ball 270 metres, but now I'm lucky to get it out there over 200 metres.

Over recent years as our friends and family grow older with us, I see some of them losing ability in these areas. An example of this would be to have to hold onto a handrail to go down a couple of steps and being quite fearful if a rail is not present.

THE GOOD NEWS

But wait, it is not all downhill gloom and doom once you have passed age thirty. What about my generation, where many are able to genuinely celebrate the idea that age seventy is now the new fifty? And deservedly so, as so many of us are into all manner of exercise activities like biking, hiking, swimming, tennis and so on. This is certainly some way ahead of most of our mums and dads.

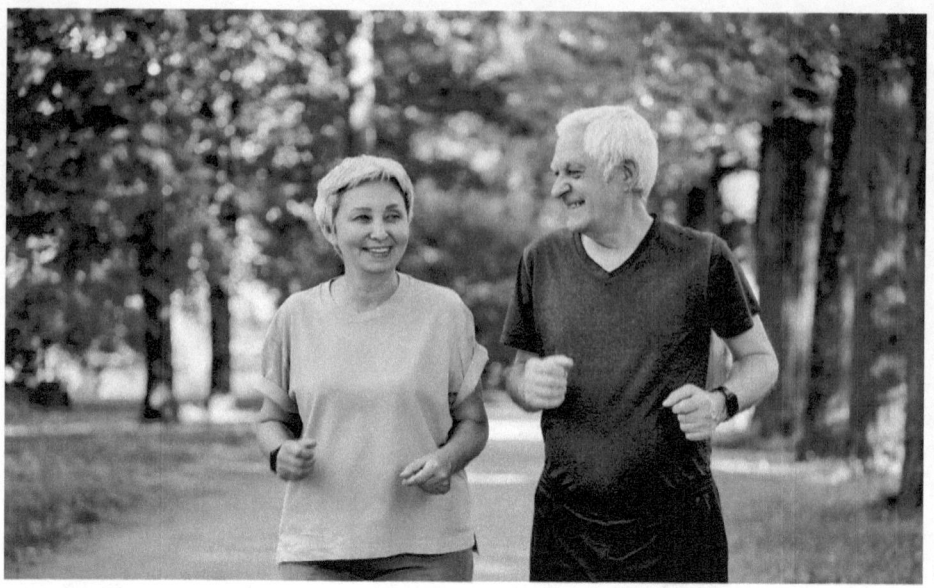

The good news is that you can delay this incremental decay by paying attention to the BAFFS: your five key cornerstones of balance, agility, cardiovascular fitness, flexibility and strength.

If you can preserve and maintain a good level of competence and fitness in each of these crucial areas, you will be giving yourself a greater chance of having a much better quality of life in your later years.

This will help to increase your healthspan years and lower your biological age. These are life-changing goals which are worth striving for.

If you have neglected some of the BAFFS, I have good news for you. Once you have embarked on a programme to improve in these areas, you will soon notice some benefits.

It is not too difficult to imagine how the combined benefits of better balance, agility, fitness, flexibility and strength will impact on your day-to-day life.

GET ALL THE BAFFS IN ONE GO

A real bonus is that many activities will provide benefits for more than one or even all of the BAFFS.

A morning's gardening, for example, might include some digging, weeding and trimming of a hedge which needs a ladder to get to the top bits.

The spade work will require some strength and get you puffing. Weeding always requires agility and flexibility, to help you to get into some of those tricky places under shrubs and flowers. And hedge trimming off a ladder includes all of these same BAFFS and has a good element of balance.

As discovered in the Langer study of housemaids, there is also another bonus. Thinking that you are getting fitter and stronger doing these household chores and leisure activities will certainly make them more enjoyable and add a motivational factor.

Walking the dog can also be a vigorous activity. Some dogs have a great knack of putting you off your stride or balance. Sudden stops and pulls in opposite directions occur, as certain smells, not always fragrant, catch the attention of their alert noses.

I will leave the rest to your imagination. There are simply heaps more activities, not actually dedicated to BAFFS, which are really effective at delivering benefits.

A reasonable level of ability in all of the BAFFS is essential.

The trick is to think about your strengths and weaknesses. Write down your various activities which provide benefits in these BAFFS areas. 'The Don't Act Your Age Challenge', which is the last chapter, will help you to assess your strengths and weaknesses and provide a BAFFS Plan to put things right.

3

MANAGING YOUR PHYSICAL HEALTH

KEY POINTS

- The number of healthspan years you are able to achieve will highly likely be in direct proportion to your ability to manage your health..
- This chapter examines how good you are, or how good you could become, at DIY in terms of managing your health.
- General practitioner – Your first line of defence against any medical complaints.
- Physiotherapist – When choosing one, I like to see some experience with sports injuries and ideally some time spent in a hospital setting helping to rehab patients.
- You can improve your DIY skills by really listening to your body. Weekend warriors can benefit by taking heed of any niggle they might feel while out playing.

- Other health professionals can include surgeons, dentists, specialists, personal trainers, chiropractors and many more.
- What should they charge? Before any appointment or treatment, always ask how much it is going to cost.
- Health insurance is relatively inexpensive in your earlier years, with both the risks to the insurer and the number of exclusions for existing conditions being lower. Over the years, as the premiums and exclusions mount, it is worth having a think about what you can do.
- Medications – If your GP tells you that you need to be on blood pressure medications, you should take up that offer.
- Being present – Anytime you are taking prescription drugs, make sure you are concentrating and being present in that moment.
- A DIY mentality can help. Making an appointment to see a doctor needs to be carefully considered. You are the one who knows best how you feel.
- As we age, a condition called sarcopenia occurs quite naturally in our muscles, causing them to lose size, strength and function.
- As you age you lose muscle mass. Muscle burns energy (calories) at twice the rate of fat. If you lose muscle mass, you will burn fewer calories, and with a slowing metabolic rate you will put on weight.
- Yoga and other stretching exercises are also vital as we age, to stretch the various elements of your skeletal system.

- Adding cardiovascular exercise to your daily routine is also crucial. Your heart, lungs and circulatory system also thrive when you get the blood pumping.
- Sitting is the new smoking – Humans are built to stand upright. Everything works better that way.

MANAGING YOUR HEALTH

If you are good at managing your health, your chances of a long and healthy life are better than someone who neglects their health.

A common thread throughout this chapter will be to examine how good you are, or how good you could become, at DIY in terms of managing your health.

Remember Tat, Sir Muir's daughter who broke her back skiing? She spent the next ten years in pain accessing various medical methods without success. Her DIY method was to head to the gym, and she managed to successfully turn things around. Traditional medicine had taken her so far and she took responsibility and applied the finishing touches herself.

It is worth repeating below Sir Muir's views on this. And I absolutely agree and will often come back to focus on this critical concept.

'It is a DIY attitude', he says, 'that can help people prevent the diseases of old age ruining their lives, or even getting a grip in the first place. An attitude that focuses on maintaining or recovering strength, stamina, suppleness and sociability whose loss many of us assume is an inevitable consequence of ageing, and so compressing the period of serious debility until as soon as possible before death.'

GENERAL PRACTITIONER

Your GP is your first line of defence against any medical complaints you may have. And arguably your most important.

I was a breech baby, in other words came out bottom or legs first, and with the umbilical cord wrapped around my neck. And not a pretty sight, being covered in eczema and a jaundiced shade of yellow.

Back in the 1940s and for a number of decades later, there was an air of pastoral care surrounding our GP practices. Home visits were the norm. I can remember cringing when the doorbell rang to announce the arrival of the doctor to give me the dreaded and painful penicillin injection in the 'you know where'.

Mum used to swear by the good doctor. Over the years I don't know how many times she told people that little Leigh here would not have been around if it hadn't been for the skill of Dr Alistair in unwrapping that cord from around my neck.

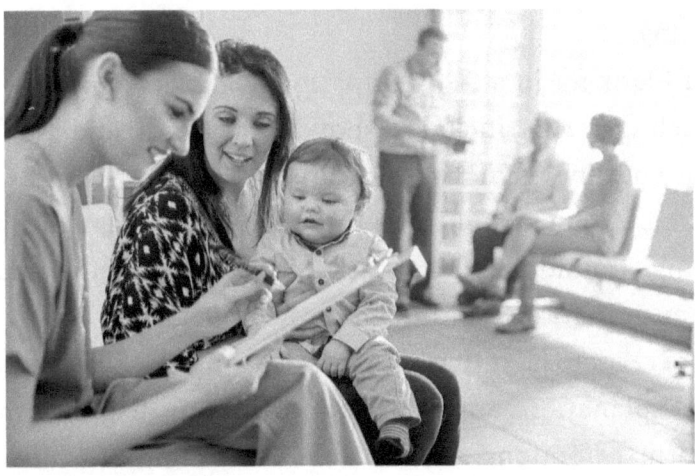

Well, how things have changed from the sedate manner in which medical practices used to be managed. These days it's all business, and doctors and nurses seem to be under constant pressure to keep up with the demands of their busy days.

One of the reasons for that could be that although we are living longer, we are sicker. Obesity, diabetes and other lifestyle diseases are now rife. The fallout from this is immense, creating far greater demand for appointments.

This creates the all-too-common problem now of not being able to see your own GP within a reasonable period of time. The only way around this is to book an appointment ahead of time and be well organised with the list of things you want to talk about. You can't always do this, and you just need to take pot luck on any given day that you have an urgent problem.

Due to my line of work helping patients with weight and diabetes issues, I have met many GPs. This is over and above the number of doctors who have attended to my own medical needs. Out of all of these GPs, I can still remember several who have stood out and that I would have also been happy to have as my own GP.

Empathy

What I look for in a GP is empathy, which is being able to relate to my feelings. This includes showing warmth and really being present as I outline what my issues are.

From here, I am looking for a thorough approach, which includes rummaging around in those dark places. For men, sometimes a digital examination, although uncomfortable, can provide immediate relief to hear that things are feeling okay up there.

Clear explanations are needed to outline any diagnosis made and what treatment options are available. For example, a model of the hip region is useful when explaining why a hip operation may be required.

I don't want any chances being taken with my health. Although my digital examination may feel alright, if my PSA is a bit high, I would rather be referred to a specialist to get their opinion than just taking a wait-and-see approach.

Hardly a day goes by without a media story about some patient's medical misadventure as the result of misdiagnosis.

Trust

You need to be able to trust your GP to go the extra mile for you.

Thinking outside the box can also pay dividends. I had had many issues over the years with bloated stomach and bowel. This had been diagnosed as irritable bowel syndrome and diverticulitis. Oddly, one day, my GP Kevin suggested that I could try Panzytrat, a supplement made from pig's pancreases. It is used to treat people whose bodies do not make enough enzymes to digest their food, such as patients with cystic fibrosis or chronic pancreatitis.

Immediately I had a massive improvement, and apart from the odd occasion these days am free from bloating and bouts of what we thought were diverticulitis symptoms. Kevin had made the connection between my symptoms and a possible pancreatic deficiency. And there is no doubt that his outside-the-box diagnosis changed my life for the better.

Communication

Communication is also important. Have other options to communicate with your GP and the practice other than only by appointments. Most practices these days have a patient portal where you can access your health records and new test results, make appointments and be able to message your GP.

Telehealth is also useful. My own practice has an app whereby I can text any symptoms I may have and receive replies from a GP. This is particularly helpful when I have a minor issue like influenza and perhaps unsure as to whether antibiotics would help.

An exchange of texts will generally provide an answer, and a script organised if required.

Second opinions

Sometimes things do not go according to plan. If you are not happy, seek a second opinion. The same goes with any other health professional you are consulting. This is part and parcel of good DIY. Do not be passive; if you think something is wrong, speak up. Seek a second opinion if you feel you are not being listened to.

I totally realise what a tough job GPs have, seeing so many patients with all manner of conditions. And patients hacking and coughing and presenting with all sorts of sometimes ghastly wounds and conditions. It does not help that they also have such a short time frame with each patient to examine, diagnose and propose the right treatment.

I understand that under all these pressures some cracks can appear. Mistakes can be life threatening, and you owe it to yourself to do some homework to ensure that you can get the best care possible.

Reputation

Ask around; if a GP has a good reputation locally, they will always be a good bet. I suppose the only downside is that with this popularity comes the problem of accessing appointments when you need them. I would say that this is a small price to pay to ensure that you get the right one.

PHYSIOTHERAPIST

Playing many sports over a long period of time, coupled with sixteen years of physical education teaching, inevitably resulted in frequent visits to physios for a wide-ranging list of injuries.

They have played a most important part in me being able to recover well and learn how to manage so many injuries.

When I have a soft-tissue injury, I will nearly always visit my physio first. This obviously changes with serious injuries like broken bones and head injuries.

With the benefit of Mr Google, it is now a simple matter to check out the experience and qualifications of local physios.

I like to see some experience with sports injuries and ideally some time spent in a hospital setting helping to rehab patients. It is helpful if they have had wide-ranging experiences in different settings.

Once again, like your GP, you need to be comfortable with your physio, know that you are being listened to, and have confidence in the treatment offered.

You want to see your physio to do some hard yards. Strong massage can be helpful in releasing different muscle groups. It can also improve blood supply and tease out any adhesions caused by injuries to tendons and other soft tissues.

Also, ideally, your physio or their practice would be also able to offer acupuncture and/or dry needling.

I had a problem with sharp nerve pains in my calf, and you could actually see the muscles vibrating. It used to catch me at most inopportune times. It was worse than cramp because of the extreme shock level of the sharp pain. I was giving a talk once to a large group of people when mid-sentence I had to stop and grab my calf. I knew some people in the audience, and even though I managed not to scream, my writhing antics caused a bit of a laugh and not a great deal of sympathy.

I had already been given some massage and heat treatment, to no avail. Once these sessions were coupled with some needling, the frequency of these episodes reduced and finally disappeared.

I also upped my magnesium supplement dosage during this time. (There will be more details about magnesium in our section on supplements.)

DIY HELPS

Once again, your DIY skills can be helpful. If you find any exercise or stretch your physio has given you causes undue pain, listen to your body and adjust or leave out this exercise, and be sure to tell the physio about it when you next see them.

I still have issues with pain in my hip and groin. Rightly diagnosed, I thought, by my physio as tightness in my medial gluteal muscle. This tightness caused the groin pain.

Exercises were aimed at strengthening areas of the hip and were fairly strenuous. My DIY mentality kicked in when I found that this condition was not improving. As I walked so often in hilly places, I decided that my hip region was already fairly strong and my flexibility was okay too. I decided to tone down the strengthening exercises and focus on stretching the gluteal muscles.

Within a week the groin pain started to disappear and stiffness in the gluteal area also improved. This injury now is practically non-existent.

You can improve your DIY skills by really listening to your body. Weekend warriors can benefit by taking heed of any niggle they might feel while out playing games like touch with their mates after a week sitting at a desk.

I am now far better at this than I used to be, although I still manage to behave like an idiot at times. My challenge is to try to live like a sixty-year-old, not like a thirty-year-old.

A few months ago, after a couple of drinks, I was egged on to do some full-on jiving and rock and roll at a function. I felt a bit of pain on the underside of my right foot and instead of backing off the high intensity, I just kept right on.

Putting my foot to the floor for the first time the next morning confirmed that, yes, I had inflamed tendons on the arch of my right foot. A few days later, after Voltaren capsules, icing and lots of stretching, thankfully I came right.

I was fortunate that this was not a more permanent injury and reasoned that I might not be so lucky next time.

SAFETY

This brings me to another really important idea: safety. The rest of this book has many ideas on different types of activities and exercises. At all times pace yourself and incrementally increase the speed and intensity of anything you are taking on. Any injury will set you back. Take care and play it safe.

OTHER HEALTH PROFESSIONALS

These can include surgeons, dentists and specialists for all different parts of your body, personal trainers, chiropractors and many more.

Similar rules apply as for GPs and physios for choosing the right one for your own personal needs.

What should they charge?

Do your homework. I am sure that there are many people around the world missing out on some of the free or heavily discounted health services that are available.

A good example of this in New Zealand is our Community Services Card which is available to people with lower incomes. Currently, a visit to a GP in Auckland will probably cost over $60, but with a Community Services Card this reduces to just $18.

Find out more at your appropriate government department's local office (in New Zealand it is Work and Income) to ensure that you are taking advantage of every opportunity like this.

Before any appointment or treatment, always ask how much it is going to cost. If you have time, and your treatment is not urgent, shop around to check that what you are paying is fair.

A friend of mine had a basal cell carcinoma on the side of his nose which needed removing and a skin graft. The local specialist clinic here quoted at least $5000. He had the operation on the Gold Coast in Australia at a reputable skin clinic at about half the cost. The operation was a success and with excellent aftercare.

SUMMARY: CHOOSING A HEALTH PROFESSIONAL

- Always check out their qualifications, experience and reputation – take nothing for granted.
- If you are not happy with your relationship with this person or their treatment, speak up or move on.
- If your condition is not improving, get a second opinion.
- And above all, always listen to your body and apply DIY methods where you see fit.

HEALTH INSURANCE

Health insurance is relatively inexpensive in your earlier years, with both the risks to the insurer and the number of exclusions for existing conditions being lower. Over the years, as the premiums and exclusions mount, it is worth considering what you can do.

One option is to increase your excess. That means that you pay the first defined amount for any procedure.

By the time we had reached a crisis point with premiums, our excess had blown out to $3000 per claim. At ages seventy-four and seventy-five, we were paying over $10,000 in excess.

Our exclusions had also mounted up. We reasoned that the obvious places for more issues to crop up would be in these exclusion areas. It seemed to be a no-brainer that if we could not get cover for these critical areas at a reasonable cost, we should cancel the health insurance.

At that stage, we had both been very well looked after by our own public health service and this also played an important part in our decision to quit.

Everybody's situation is different. If you are thinking about taking up or terminating health insurance, take your time and weigh up all the pros and cons.

In hindsight, we would now probably have talked to our GP about our health, the costs and what they thought. To date we have been fortunate to not have had any serious illnesses or accidents and have saved over $100,000 in premiums.

MEDICATIONS

My sister Kaye had a quite serious stroke when she was eighty. This affected her mobility, and she was learning to walk again. I remember while helping her into a wheelchair, she looked up at me with very sad eyes, and said, 'What a bloody circus.' She usually never swore.

It turned out that her GP had been keen for her to go on blood-pressure medication. Despite continued high BP readings, she still had turned down this request a number of times.

The stroke was a bitter pill to swallow for her (pun intended), knowing that it probably could have been averted if she had only listened and acted on her GP's advice.

I also found out later there had been some opinions expressed by her family which may have affected Kaye's decision. If you have a loved one who is being offered possibly life-saving orthodox medical advice, keep your own alternative views to yourself.

Shortly after moving into a retirement village, Kaye had a rectal bleed which proved to be a bridge too far. She decided to seek no further medical help and sadly passed away in a local hospice about a month later.

Some years before this, when I was in my early sixties, my same GP Kevin was telling me that on the back of some high blood pressure readings it was time to start taking BP medication. Of course, I remonstrated with him that they weren't that high. He kept at it, and after drawing me some graphic pictures on the life-changing effects of strokes, I gave in.

You see, back then I felt invincible. How could anything go wrong? I was a classic case of death denial, and thank goodness Kevin persevered and had me start taking those little white pills.

Prescription reviews

Over the years, having had the rest home experience and consultancies with patients, I have seen lots of lists of medications. In most cases, all of these medications are necessary to help with various conditions. In others, I believe that they have accumulated over a number of years and have never been reviewed.

An elderly close relation was about to travel to the UK, and we thought that he was just too confused and unsteady to travel alone. A change of GP and a review of his meds revealed that many of them were simply not relevant and necessary. Within a week on his reduced meds intake, he almost magically gained clarity of mind and his balance improved quite dramatically.

Off he flew to England and arrived back a month later in great spirits and full of stories.

I think the message is quite clear. It is really important to review your medications with your GP from time to time.

Side-effects

Many of us will check out medications on the internet, and although this can be helpful, sometimes the long lists of side-effects can be very scary. It is important to note, however, that these are side-effects taken from a very large sample of people.

If a medication is prescribed, you are better to try it out than think you know better than your doctor and not take it. If after taking the medication you do have side-effects, a plan B will be required.

And the reverse can also apply. I was suffering from a painful neural condition in the pelvic floor. After a battery of tests, no clear diagnosis was able to be made.

My GP at the time would not prescribe a neuromuscular drug

which seemed to be quite appropriate for my condition. (I discuss this more fully later in the book.)

In hindsight I should have been more insistent. I had sought other opinions informally which concurred with mine, but I did not push my case enough. Probably the right course of action would have been to seek a second opinion.

This once again underlines the importance of both getting a second opinion and acting on it if you think it is right. And be a 'squeaky wheel' if you feel that you are not being listened to.

Being present

Anytime you are taking prescription drugs, make sure you are concentrating and being present in that moment. If you are distracted by other matters and not singularly focused, you may have difficulty remembering whether you took them.

Once you start taking any medication, it is vital that you are compliant with the instructions on the label. And be consistent by taking the recommended dose, and at the right time.

You need to see your GP or pharmacist if you get to a stage where you are taking multiple drugs and get confused at all about when you have taken them last. They will set you up with a pill organiser like a weekly blister pack.

In summary, if a GP recommends that you take a medication, take it. If you are not happy with this decision or any other aspect of your care, get a second opinion. If the number of drugs you take is growing, initiate a review with your GP about this. If you get confused about when and what you have taken, get a pill organiser system.

DIY MENTALITY

A DIY mentality can help. You do need to take some responsibility for your health yourself. Making an appointment to see a doctor needs to be carefully considered. You are the one who knows best how you feel. Do I really need to go to my GP about this? Am I becoming part of the 'worried well', or perhaps even a hypochondriac?

I will not comment on specific drugs and their use, as this is best left to the professionals. One thing I will say, though, is that you don't need to be too hard on yourself when it comes to dealing with pain.

I know people who are so staunch when it comes to even taking paracetamol. Inflammation is often a root cause of pain and really stresses body tissues. You are better to take an anti-inflammatory tablet, as prescribed by your doctor, to ease the pain than cause unnecessary ongoing stress to your body and yourself. Obviously if the pain continues, you should seek medical advice.

Managing your health comes down to managing two broad categories: physical health and mental health. We will take a look at the former first.

YOUR PHYSICAL HEALTH

We have already covered the importance of maintaining cardiovascular fitness, strength, balance and flexibility. All of these vital areas rely heavily on the ability of your muscles, cartilage, tendons and ligaments to be able to cope with the stresses of actually being capable in all of these areas.

I now want to drill down into some of these physical aspects in more detail.

The crucial components of your skeletal system are muscles, tendons, ligaments and cartilage. Muscles are attached to bone by tendons, ligaments attach bone to bone in joints, and the cartilage helps to cushion bone on bone in joints.

Weight/resistance training

As we age, a scary condition called sarcopenia occurs quite naturally in our muscles. This means our muscles lose size, strength and function.

Our tendons and ligaments lose collagen, so they become weakened and lose flexibility. And the cushioning cartilage loses fluid and becomes less effective. It sometimes fails completely, creating a bone-on-bone situation in our joints.

The good news is that weight and/or resistance training which puts stress on all parts of our skeletal system can slow down and improve sarcopenia and deterioration in our tendons, ligaments and cartilage.

Resistance training includes working with stretchy bands, weights or self-resistance exercises which pit muscle against muscle.

Any other activity which involves your muscles being worked against some sort of resistance will help, as in gardening, housework, cycling and climbing stairs.

Despite maintaining the same lifestyle, people often wonder why they put on weight as they age. As you age, as we have just discussed, you lose muscle mass. Muscle burns energy (calories) at twice the rate of fat. If you lose muscle mass, you will burn fewer calories, and with a slowing metabolic rate you will put on weight. This is another great reason to regularly work out with weights or some other form of resistance training.

Yoga and other stretching exercises are also vital as we age, to stretch the various elements of our skeletal system.

Unless your muscles, joints, tendons, ligaments and cartilage have deteriorated beyond a point of no return, you will always gain benefits by carrying out these various exercises. These benefits of increasing muscle strength and skeletal flexibility are well worth striving for to slow down the ageing process and increase your healthspan years.

Cardiovascular exercise

Adding cardiovascular exercise to your daily routine is also crucial. Your heart, lungs and circulatory system also thrive when you get the blood pumping through all the different vessels. This can reduce the chance of having a stroke, heart attack, high blood pressure, diabetes and other life-limiting medical events and conditions.

Sleep

You spend about one third of your life sleeping, and seven to nine hours of sleep a night is essential for you to have continued good health.

A full night's sleep helps to support healthy brain function and overall physical health.

If you regularly have trouble sleeping and endure restless nights, you are likely to have memory, focus, mood and immune system issues. If these are long-term problems, you are more likely to prematurely suffer a chronic illness. In this case it is vital that you should contact your GP to work through the possible issues and find a solution.

Breathing

Most of us are fortunate that we can just take breathing for granted; it just happens day in day out. But asthmatics and people with other lung issues often struggle to get enough air into their lungs and need to use nebulisers and other medications.

Unknowingly, many of us become regular shallow chest

breathers and often breathe through our mouth. This can happen in situations where you are stressed or even simply concentrating on one or other task you are involved with. This can lead to a lack of oxygen to our lungs, circulatory system and other bodily tissues. In some cases, it can elevate stress levels and cause panic attacks.

I am guilty of shallow breathing, particularly when I am writing, and I need to become more aware of this. I try to use my diaphragm more. This is a muscle under the lungs which helps to pull more air into the lungs.

I have little expertise in this important area and decided to just mention breathing in my book to raise awareness of this very common shallow-breathing issue.

If you do have breathing issues, there are plenty of experts around who can help. Various methods like Buteyko (which aims to reduce over-breathing and promotes nasal breathing) are effective in helping you to improve any issues you may have.

Standing

Sitting is the new smoking. I often hear people talk about the two big gym sessions they go to a week, or the big tramp that they go on in the weekend. Twice or three times a week full-on efforts are no doubt good for your fitness. Much of these benefits are lost if the remaining four or five days are spent sitting at a desk.

Humans are built to stand upright. Everything works better that way. *Your heart, cardiovascular system and other organs function more efficiently when you are standing.*

Long periods of sitting can lead to the weakening of the large leg and gluteal (bum) muscles. The same can happen with your hip and back muscles and will be likely to affect your posture. Pain and stiffness in your shoulders can also be experienced.

Even your digestion will not be as efficient, and sedentary

workers have far higher rates of anxiety and depression than more active people.

Break up long periods of sitting with regular breaks to get yourself moving in some way and, ideally, with your heart rate up. There are many ways of doing this, and this is discussed more fully later in the Don't Act Your Age Challenge, and it includes a number of examples for you to follow.

The bottom line: some form of regular daily exercise is the key.

ARCH JELLEY'S STORY

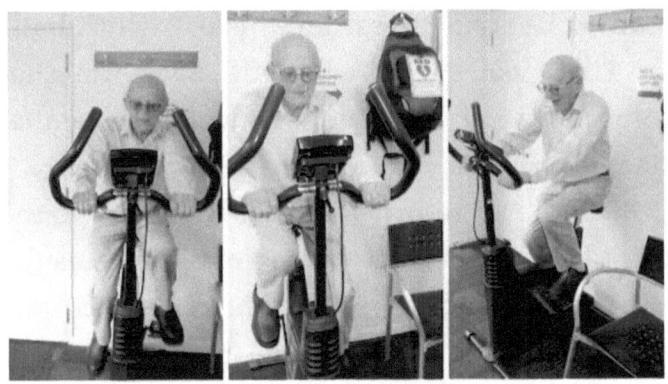

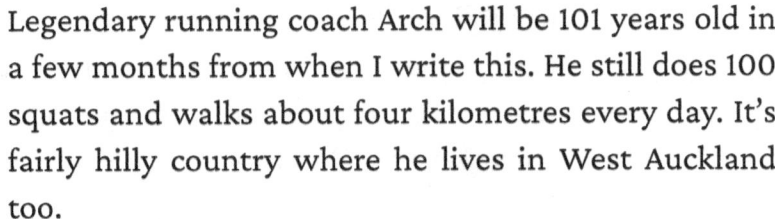

Legendary running coach Arch will be 101 years old in a few months from when I write this. He still does 100 squats and walks about four kilometres every day. It's fairly hilly country where he lives in West Auckland too.

He cuts himself a bit of slack these days and stopped running up the three flights of stairs to his apartment when he was ninety-two. Sitting in his chair opposite me, he still looks to be in his seventies and is in really good shape.

As he sits in his chair, one ankle rests comfortably above the knee of his other leg. I surreptitiously do the same and try for the same upper leg angle. I find this quite difficult; he still has very good hip flexibility.

I'm also impressed when Arch gets up out of his chair in one fluid movement with absolutely no sign of any stiffness.

Born in Dunedin in August 1922, Arch's first memory is that of falling off a very small merry-go-round while trying to retrieve his hat which had fallen off. This was at the South Seas International Exhibition in Dunedin and was held in November 1926 when he was four years old.

His father, a returned soldier who was wounded at Gallipoli, was a small businessman in the suburb of Mornington. Sadly, his father's brother died at Passchendaele in 1917 at the age of twenty-one.

'We were hard up, as most people were in those Depression years, but we never felt deprived.'

His teacher Bill Wallace was a veteran of twenty-five years' teaching at the Mornington School and soccer was his game. His popularity meant that the kids all played soccer too. This was most unusual for a rugby-mad country.

Arch put this right when he went to Otago Boys High School, and when he was seventeen he was the captain of the under eight stone (fifty kg) rugby team. Obviously small in stature, for most of his adult life he was sixty-three kilos and is still about the same weight today.

He was only about thirty kilos when he went to high school and was invited to join the gymnastic squad, telling me that his only real qualification was his small size. The ten smallest third formers were usually invited to become members of the squad. After applying himself diligently, but possessing only average talent, he became the school gymnastic champion in his last year at school.

As I listen to Arch tell his story, I am amazed at his razor-sharp memory, recalling events and people from many decades earlier. He possesses a wonderfully quirky sense of humour to go with this. He holds up his right hand and I can see that the tip of his fourth finger is missing.

'My older brother and I were trying to cut the lawn. He had hedge-clippers and I had a large pair of scissors. I got too close to the hedge-clippers and the top joint of my finger was almost sliced off.' I didn't ask him what the size of the lawn was. He remembered his father cutting the remaining thread of tissue holding the fingertip and depositing it in a hole in the garden.

With his father he then walked up to the terminus, took the cable car to the city and then the electric tram along Princes Street. A week in hospital followed to treat the finger and keep an eye on the healing. We both agree that these days a better outcome would have probably resulted.

When Arch left school he joined the Survey Department as a cadet. Shortly after this at age eighteen he and his mate Alan MacLauchlan were conscripted into the Scottish Regiment, but the next year they applied for entry into the navy's Scheme B. This was for those who may have the potential to become naval officers.

They were posted to HMS *Tamaki* in Auckland and were then sent on final leave before sailing for England on the *Ruahine* via the Panama Canal and New York. Arch celebrated his twenty-first in Jack Dempsey's bar in New York.

The fifty New Zealanders in Scheme B then trained at HMS *Ganges* at Shotley Gate in England for three months, before Arch was posted as an Ordinary Seaman to HMS *Bermuda* in November 1943. 'There were fifty New Zealanders in training at *Ganges* and there is only one still alive and he's sitting right opposite you.' I could work that one out.

The *Bermuda* left Scapa Flow and then joined a convoy just off Reykjavik in Iceland before proceeding to Kola Peninsula, north of Murmansk in the Soviet Union.. Luckily, they struck really bad weather with low cloud which protected them from detection from German aircraft and submarines.

Arch was three or four decks down in the bowels of the ship. 'I was in the control room of the high-angle guns, and although snug and warm, reflected at times that we would have no show getting out if we were badly hit.

'There were some interesting guys on the Bermuda and one of these was Bruce Mason.' Bruce became a well-known New Zealand playwright whose most famous work was *The End of the Golden Weather*. They got lucky again, leaving Kola as the weather was rough and the convoy and escorts arrived back in the UK unscathed.

Arch was among those sent to King Alfred in Hove to undergo an officers' training course. After being commissioned, he was posted to Greenwich to a finishing school for officers to teach them the correct demeanour and the like. Denis Glover, who later became a famous New Zealand poet, pithily remarked, 'We're not gentlemen, we're New Zealanders.'

For some unaccountable reason which Arch to this day cannot explain, he opted for submarines when asked what branch he fancied. And so off to Blyth on the Northumberland coast for more training of the underwater variety, from which he emerged as a Navigator or Gunnery/ Torpedo Officer on coastal submarines.

After the war in November 1945 Arch and his older brother Charlie, who was in the Fleet Air Arm, left Southampton on their way back home, but halfway across the Bay of Biscay they had to turn back because a turbine had broken down.

They both spent the next few weeks in Paris and Brussels before once again setting sail for New Zealand. Arch and Charlie had bought a book on the card game of bridge. After swotting it up for a while, they entered a competition and came second without knowing much about the game. This was a clear sign of things to come.

On their way back to Dunedin, Arch, Charles and his new girlfriend attended a family gathering in Christchurch. Arch asked his brother who the young fellow was who seemed to know a lot about our family.

'Jesus Christ Arch, that's your brother Stan!' Much laughter and celebration followed. It turned out that young Stan had grown a fair bit in the three years that he had been away. Arch wryly commented, 'Even on the Jelley scale.'

Back home in Dunedin he resigned from the Survey Department and enrolled in a two-year teachers' college course and to study for a BA. at Otago University. A busy and enjoyable life followed. He managed to fit some cricket in too when at college. 'I remember being hit to all corners of the ground at a practice session by the famous cricket test batsman Bert Sutcliffe.'

After qualifying at Dunedin Teachers' College, he applied for the nearest sole-charge school to Dunedin. This turned out to be a tiny school, Rata-iti, nearly a thousand kilometres by road and up in the North Island, in the Rangitikei area, near Hunterville.

As a single man, Arch boarded with different families when he taught at Rata-iti School. Arch had moved to a new place four or five miles from the school and his powers of endurance and strength were about to be tested to the limit.

On an initial run of discovery in his newfound area, he got lost in the mist in what was very hilly country. It was winter and very cold; Arch had on only shorts and a singlet. It turned out to be a long run of fifteen hours.

The *Wanganui Chronicle*'s headline was, 'Unexpected Marathon'. To keep warm, he ran around the top of a large hill most of the night. It is not surprising that he had a few falls in the dark.

'Luckily, I was pretty fit and strong. About seven in the morning the mist had cleared and I jogged down to a red-roofed house in the valley below. I knocked on the door and a Māori lady opened it and said, "Oh good morning," almost as if she had been expecting me. There was no school that day.

'The next day at school, Kelvin our school monitor, who was about as tall as I was, lit the fire. I sat huddled by this fire as I just could not get warm.

'Luckily our Physical Education adviser, Don Beard, turned up and said, "Stay where you are Arch, I'll teach the school today,' and I remained right by the fire all day. It was fortunate that Arch had been tough and resilient as it sounds like his core temperature had got very low, indicating a close call with hypothermia.

Don Beard, his saviour on that day, went on to become a test cricketer and featured in New Zealand's first test cricket win against the West Indies in 1956.

Arch's next move was in 1952 to the Tawa School in

Wellington where he met Rachel who was also teaching at the school, and the next year they were married. Arch said that this was a turning point for him. He found her directness somewhat disconcerting at first but soon started looking at the world in a different light. Any problem was met head on and a solution found. Anything was achievable.

In 1956 Rachel's brother Doug resigned as a teacher and went to the States to study chiropractic. Rachel's mother became down in the dumps as she was losing her only son.

Rachel became pregnant later in 1956. The pregnancy had been a planned operation as Rachel had felt her mother needed something more tangible to replace her only son. Arch didn't need much encouragement before he collaborated with Rachel in her devious plan.

In December 1957 Arch and Rachel decided that it was time for a change and looked at the respective house prices in Wellington and Auckland. Surprisingly, Auckland houses were less expensive, which is certainly not the case today. After a short spell living with Rachel's estranged father in Auckland, they bought a house in Mt Albert in which they stayed for the next twenty-seven years. During this time they had three children, Su, Martin and Rocky.

Arch's teaching career blossomed and after a number of headships including Napier Street School in Freeman's Bay, he became the foundation principal of Sunnybrae Normal School on Auckland's North Shore.

Arch recalls dabbling with running coaching in his Dunedin years, where he had organised a locality scheme which operated across the city for members of the Mornington club. They all used a common training schedule that he had prepared.

'Although our club was a small one, we still managed to win a number of provincial titles.' Arch's two brothers were also into athletics and whichever club they were in they always made significant contributions.

In the Akaroa Relay in 1960, the three brothers, ran a 'race within a race', when they all ran the same leg for their respective teams. At that time, they were all captains of their respective clubs.

His athletics coaching career began in earnest in 1959 when he joined the Owairaka Athletics club. In the 1960s there were two distinct groups that trained in the famed Waitakere Ranges. This era signalled a hugely significant time in world middle and long-distance running history initiated by legendary coach Arthur Lydiard.

Arthur had an established group which included famous names like Murray Halberg, Peter Snell, Barry Magee and Bill Baillie. They all went on to win Olympic medals or set world records. Peter Snell is now recognised as perhaps one of the greatest ever 800-metre runners.

'Bruce Stuart was the first runner I coached in Auckland. Although Bruce was not academically inclined, he compiled a lengthy record of life experiences. I recorded what he told me and his exact words are in a booklet which is a valuable primary source on Bruce's life.

'Formerly coached by Arthur, he wouldn't do as he was told and was thrown out of Arthur's squad and came to me. Bruce usually took my advice, and I remember the extraordinary amounts of tea and orange juice he consumed after our weekly twenty-two mile runs round the Waitakeres. We didn't realise at the time that this was possibly a sign that he was pre-diabetic. Sadly, he succumbed to diabetes at a relatively early age.'

Arch recalls training a large enthusiastic group of mostly club runners who enjoyed their training and racing, with many becoming lifelong friends. The first athletes to reach international class in Arch's group were Neville Scott, a recovering alcoholic who was a brilliant runner, and Ian Studd who won the bronze medal in the 1500 metres at the 1966 Empire Games in Jamaica.

One night in Manurewa, Neville had an opportunity to defeat Halberg, a man possessing incredible resolve and determination. Neville simply ran away from Halberg in the early stages of the 5000 metres event, but Halberg overtook him and won the race. Unaccountably, Neville had taken his track shoes off a few minutes before the start of the race and the soles of his bare feet were soon in a terrible mess, and he paid the penalty for a very bad decision.

In the late 1960s a tall rangy young fellow came up

to Arch at a Hobsonville cross-country meeting and told him that he had been beaten for the first time in a cross-country race. The tall rangy fellow was John Walker.

Arch told him that everybody gets beaten sooner or later and asked him what his training regime was. His answer was that he did no training and only ran on race days. Arch told him that the guy that beat him, Stitch McRae, ran about ninety miles a week on a planned schedule and was trained by well-known coach Don MacFarquhar.

Arch gave him a six-week training schedule and few weeks later he won the Auckland junior cross-country championships, but he was defeated in the NZ Junior championships a few weeks later. Arch coached John for a while, but they eventually lost touch.

In 1971, John, now a senior, made the final in the 800 metres in the national championships, but came last in the final. In August 1971 John approached Arch to see if he would consider coaching him again and said this time he would work really hard at it. 'Initially I thought that he was okay as a runner but never thought he would become the best middle-distance runner in the world.'

This all changed when John easily beat Dick Quax over 800 metres at a big meeting in Tauranga in a personal best time on 1 January 1972. He had already done his training and ran in borrowed gear. Even though Dick's best distance was 5000 metres or longer, Arch was so impressed that he wrote to the New Zealand selectors about John.

Arch wrote that John was big, strong and fast, had a good temperament and might even surpass Peter Snell's records. He also sent a similar letter to *The Wellington Sports Post* and won the letter of the week. An Art Union ticket was the prize, which Arch wryly reflects did not win any money.

In 1972 John had an easy win in the national 800 metres championships in Hamilton but was later defeated by All Black winger Bruce Hunter in what was an Olympic trial for Munich. Neither John nor Bruce made the Olympic team.

In Vancouver the following year John was not pleased when not allowed to run in the A Grade mile, and Dick Quax was upset by some remark that John made about this race and said to John, 'Walker, you'll never make a runner's a***hole.' John won the B grade race in 3:58.

Dick and John were soon reconciled and Dick and Rod Dixon took John with them on a tour of Europe. They pulled strings to get this unknown runner into races, in which he did quite well. Although John arrived home exhausted, rubbing shoulders with and racing against these world-class runners had been an invaluable experience.

Arch recalls the build-up to the 1500 metres final at the Commonwealth Games in Christchurch in 1974. John was staying out of the village at this stage at his brother Stan's place in Christchurch.

'We played backyard cricket and John was in for ages hunched over this really small bat. We were concerned when he woke up the next day with a stiff back just a day before the final. We went for a run to help loosen this up and laughed when some kid yelled out, "Who do you think you are, Olympians?"

'We wondered whether or not the kid was watching TV the next day when both Filbert Bayi and John broke the world record in the 1500 metres. Filbert won by a couple of metres and I remember looking at my watch to see in amazement that they had both broken the world record.

'I'm a fairly quiet coach normally, but on this occasion I apparently jumped up on my seat shouting, "It's a world record, it's a world record!" I've no recollection of this, but brother Stan assured me that this is what I did.

'Most critics were not surprised at Bayi's victory but could not credit that John could also break the world record and reduce his best time by six seconds. [American athlete] Marty Liquori said, "Bayi, yes, but Walker, no way." Liquori was saying that John's phenomenal improvement could not have occurred naturally. How wrong he was!'

On 12 August 1975 John ran in a mile race in Gothenburg in Sweden and not only smashed Filbert Bayi's world record but also became the first person to run under the magical 3:50. Rod Dixon and journalist Ivan Agnew were there and were the first to congratulate him. It was 13 August in New Zealand,

Arch's birthday. What a marvellous birthday present for the coach!

From that day on, John's life changed and he was eagerly sought by promoters worldwide.

Prior to the 1976 Olympics in Montreal, John and Arch headed off to Scandinavia for some warm-up races with other members of the New Zealand Olympic team. In one of these races, John ran the 2000 metres distance in an incredible time. He took over four seconds off the world record, perhaps his greatest ever race.

At Montreal he ran a disappointing race in the 800 metres, though Arch was rather relieved as there is no way he wanted John to compete in two finals. A reporter asked him if he was disappointed with his defeat. John replied, 'Well, not really. I had a far bigger disappointment that night when my coach beat me at snooker for the very first time.'

On the 1500 metres final day, Arch and John had a two-hour snooze before the race. Arch commented that sharing a room with John had some limitations. He had so much gear that Arch was restricted to a very small area.

Filbert Bayi, his main rival, was out with malaria and without a pacemaker the pace was really too slow for John. He went to the front early in the last lap and, just outlasting the rest, threw his arms into the air in celebration just before the line. John became one of the greatest middle-distance runners of all time.

He became both the first to run the mile in under

3:50 and to run 100 sub-four-minute miles. He was knighted in 2009 for his services to athletics and the community.

Arch and John remain great friends and see each other regularly. I ask Arch whether or not they talk about that Olympic gold, and he replied in the negative, as they probably have a great many other things to talk about.

Apart from John, Arch trained dozens of top-class athletes and coached and managed many New Zealand teams to the Olympic Games and World Championships. He was also involved as an administrator and was awarded a CNZM and an OBE for his services to athletics and to bridge.

More recently in 2024 at the age of 102, with many thinking that this was well overdue, Arch was awarded a life membership of Athletics New Zealand.

Rachel and Arch were great friends with David and Jean Metzger, and they travelled widely together. Arch and Jean played in bridge tournaments wherever possible, while the other two would happily check out the local tourist spots and antique shops.

In 2000, both David and Rachel died within six months of each other. Arch and Jean remained good friends and continued to play bridge together, and in 2002 they were married.

To avoid any fuss, they ended up not telling their children until after the event − not a universally popular decision. There seemed to be confusion about whether or not Arch even proposed to Jean, and she is fairly certain he will not go down in history as one of the great romantics. He says he's the pragmatic type, whatever that means.

They have lived happily ever since in their apartment at The Pinesong Retirement Village in Green Bay, Auckland. Arch says he has been doubly blessed in that Rachel and Jean have put up with his obsessions and supported him in every possible way.

Arch said that Jean had one trait which was well nigh impossible to eradicate. This was her daily habit of picking up anything left lying on the floor which was obviously not in its proper place. This often meant that items Arch had deliberately placed on the floor as a reminder for something had vanished without trace.

I was interested in digging a bit more deeply into what really makes this great man tick. 'Well, I think really that I am a bit quiet and introverted. My teaching style was such that I was pretty relaxed and I enjoyed my various teaching experiences.

'When I was a principal I encouraged everyone to participate, irrespective of their seniority. At Sunnybrae and at Napier Street, I thought most of the teachers were better classroom teachers than I ever was. I took a great interest in all my teachers and athletes and actually coaching is all about helping people to find their own way, and their own solutions.'

I told Arch that I had heard a rumour that he could be a bit obsessive. Jean had told me earlier that he had over 300 books on bridge. 'I think there might be a bit of truth in that and I think I did have three hundred and fifty bridge books at one stage, before I gave about half of them to members of our bridge club.

'I had been interested in the game of bridge since just after the war and one day in 1991 Rachel had said to me, why didn't I join the Mt Albert Bridge Club and learn to play bridge properly.' After Arch had consulted some notes from his brother, who had become a bridge teacher, he went down to the bridge club and has been playing bridge ever since.

He now thinks bridge is the greatest game ever devised as it can be played by anyone of any age, any gender, size, or race and at any time. It can also be played online. As well as playing at the club twice a week Arch plays bridge online about once a week.

He sometimes plays against Sybil who is also a centenarian and whose son Michael was a world champion a few years ago. Somerset Maugham said of bridge, 'In fact when all else fails – sport, love, ambition – bridge remains a solace and an entertainment.'

Arch has written a number of booklets on the subject and designed his own bridge system called 'Archway Precision'. He didn't choose the title which Jean still considers rather pretentious.

Arch took up bowls when he was eighty years old and started off as a junior. Anybody is classified as a junior irrespective of age and who has been playing for less than five years. He was a member of two teams that won Auckland titles and was also a member of the

Auckland Development squad until it was discovered how old he was.

SUMMING UP ARCH

When Arch's 100th was celebrated at the bridge club, Mary, the club director, said with tongue in cheek that there were three explanations for Arch's longevity:

First: Exercise and brain power!
Second: He was dropped here from outer space!
Third: He was not born in 1922 but in 1942.

If I didn't know what Arch's real age was, I would have put him as being twenty to thirty years younger. A closer look at how he has achieved this provides many clues as to how to have a biological age way below your actual age.

Attitude – Always positive and optimistic, he keeps a cool head under pressure, and this has always led to a low-stress lifestyle. The ability to train many top athletes including an all-time great, and surviving the rigours of a long and successful teaching career, are also testament to this great attitude. And add to this, earlier on, his engagement in the Second World War.

Despite being a high achiever in a number of fields, this modest and kind man with a quirky sense of humour would not be one to 'sweat the small stuff'.

A natural leader, he managed to get the best out of his teachers and runners and took a keen interest in them all. He would prefer to take a look at himself first if they were not doing that well.

Arch has a philosophy based on 'use the difficulty', a phrase popularised by actor Michael Caine. As a young actor Michael was waiting to come on stage, when his entrance was blocked by a chair thrown in his path. He appealed to the director who replied, 'Use the difficulty. If it's a tragedy, smash the chair and if it's a comedy, fall over it.'

By this he meant that however bad the situation appears, something positive and good can usually emerge. Jean and Arch recently sold their car and are now without wheels, meaning that their self-dependence is threatened to a certain extent. However, without a car they are now better off financially and their fitness has improved because they are both walking greater distances each day. They've used the difficulty.

A healthy weight and life – It is no surprise that Jean and Arch have porridge for breakfast and eat a well-balanced diet. A couple of beers the odd time in earlier life, but he now no longer drinks alcohol.

Physical health – Extremely fit all his life, he still follows a fairly rigorous daily schedule of about a four-kilometre walk and 100 squats.

With regard to the BAFFS five areas of the physical foundation blocks, he has no weaknesses.

- Balance – He can stand on one leg and on tiptoes. Although he has one hand lightly resting on the handrail, he easily walks up and down stairs.
- Agility – The key to having good agility revolves around your ability to easily move your feet in different directions. Arch still walks at a reasonable pace and some of his walks are quite hilly.

- He can easily get down and up off the floor but thinks he would now struggle to do a squat thrust (burpee).
- Fitness – Daily walks, the odd flight of stairs and some sessions on his stationary bike ensure a good level of cardiovascular fitness.
- Flexibility – Arch admits to not being a great one to stretch during his life and can touch his toes with some difficulty. Nonetheless, he does not often get stiff and sore and has no ongoing pain.
- Strength – The ability to do multiple squats indicates a very good level of core strength.

Purpose – He always has some sort of project on the go. With eight children and a large extended family between them, Arch and Jean are closely connected to their family and friends daily.

He retains internet, email, Zoom and mobile phone connections, while a Garmin watch helps him to keep track of his heart rate, the kilometres he walks and how various athletes are doing around the world.

Arch expertly edited a large part of this draft story that I sent him earlier on.

Mental capacity – I rate this as unbelievable. His recollection of dates, names, athletics times, events and other stuff from up to ninety years ago is simply phenomenal.

In sum – Arch's two brothers lived until age ninety-five and his 'little' sister is still going strong at ninety. He is following this same longevity trend which is certainly a strong genetic advantage.

Along the way he has had three broken bones to deal with, all sports related. He had a frontal craniotomy for meningioma in 2004, a heart valve replaced in 2003, and a full knee replacement 2020. He calls the brain operation his 'brain transplant' and remembers missing a whole week of bridge because of it.

Fortunately, none of these proved to be life-threatening and Arch acknowledges that he has had some luck along the way.

We have already talked about his positive attitude, generosity and constantly having purpose to his life. Being a headmaster and coach of many champion athletes, including one legendary one, could have proved to be a very stressful life. Arch's relaxed, inclusive approach ensured that his stress levels were more often than not well under control. He is not prone to self-absorption and his quirky sense of humour reflects the fact that he does not take himself and life too seriously.

He always walked the talk and the daily disciplines that he applied to his athletes were followed by the man himself. Athletes train daily and he has carried this regime on to this day, albeit in a far more relaxed and sedate manner.

Arch has taken warfarin, a blood thinner, since his heart-valve replacement seven or eight years ago. He takes no other medication.

His abilities in all of the five physical criteria, balance, agility, fitness, flexibility and strength, are still at a level far superior to many people decades younger.

Mentally he is still amazing and pursuits like genealogy and bridge certainly help to retain this mental edge.

What a pleasure and privilege it has been to meet Arch and Jean and many thanks for sharing your wonderful life story with us.

4
MANAGING YOUR MENTAL HEALTH

KEY POINTS

- In this chapter I try to cover some of the concepts that have worked well for me to keep me on top of things mentally.
- 'Life stinks. And the sooner you accept this, the better off you'll be.' We need to embrace reality, have a higher level of self-understanding, and become a much more sensitive and happy person.
- The key is to accept the hard things and do away with the delusion that your life will be a straight line of pleasant experiences.
- Don't sweat the small stuff... when you let go of your expectations and accept life as it is – you're free.
- Be grateful – Our busy lives with all their different

challenges will often get in the road of the basic things in life that we love and should be grateful for.
- Beware of issues with computers and the like such as long periods of sitting, neck and sight issues, and social media and smartphone addictions.
- If you regularly feel out of sorts mentally and generally unhappy with your life, seek help.
- Accept that life is going to throw you many curveballs and you just need to get on and deal with them.

FACING CHALLENGES, EMBRACING REALITY

One of the best bits of advice I ever received came from a book called *The Road Less Travelled* by M. Scott Peck. This is a very influential work written over twenty-five years ago by this eminent psychiatrist. It deals with helping to confront and solve problems. In a similar way to denial of death, we often simply try to avoid some of these issues and inevitably they will get worse.

This book shows you how to embrace reality, have a higher level of self-understanding, and become a much more sensitive and happy person.

The publishers claim that *The Road Less Travelled* has changed many lives for the better. I would have to agree.

This piece of good advice was along the lines of this summary about the book, 'Let's not mince words: life stinks. And the sooner you accept this, the better off you'll be.'

Although this is a bit over the top, it obviously means that your life will present with many different problems and challenges for you to face. The key is to accept this and do away with the delusion that your life will be a straight line of pleasant experiences. *If you can dispense with the rose-tinted spectacles and be ready for the challenges ahead, whatever they may be, you are halfway to solving them.* As it says in the great lyric from The Moody Blues song 'In the Beginning', 'Face piles of trials with smiles.'

The second best bit of advice that I have received is *'Don't sweat the small stuff...and it's all small stuff.* When you let go of your expectations, when you accept life as it is, you're free. To hold on is to be serious and uptight. To let go is to lighten up.'

This is from the book, *Don't Sweat the Small Stuff* by Richard Carlson and is a useful extension to the first idea about accepting life's ups and downs.

And so, logically, if you can achieve both states of mind, you will accept that 'shit happens', ignore the small stuff and get onto dealing with the big stuff.

What is small stuff? Well, this is going to vary according to your age, sex, vocation, social and sporting interests and so on.

For instance, a triple bogey to finish off a round for a keen golfer may be seen as small stuff. This event would become rather more highly magnified if this had stuffed up the golfer's chance of breaking eighty for the first time. Any golfer, me included, would naturally feel disappointed by this. The key here is: for how long.

You will get flat tyres, blocked toilets, inclement weather, late trains, late friends, be late yourself, get criticised and the list is infinite. This is all small stuff; no one has died or become critically injured. You have not lost your job or suffered crippling financial loss.

I see so many people waste so much time moaning and agonising over small stuff. If it's something like the weather which you can't change, you're wasting your time moaning about it. If it's something you can't control, forget about it. If it's something that you can control, deal with it at your first opportunity.

If you have friends who are always moaning and negative about almost everything, they can drag you down too. If you can, try to talk to them about this. If they are not receptive to your suggestions, spend less time with them.

All of these concepts above are basic traits of human nature. Just remember that you have a choice as to which pathway you wish to go down. Choose wisely.

BEING GRATEFUL

Our busy lives with all their challenges will often get in the road of the basic things in life that we love and should be grateful for.

Gratitude is an attitude. Being grateful is a powerful antidote to all things negative in your life. Highlighting all of your positives and the things you love feels great.

I vividly remember my thought patterns immediately after being diagnosed with a melanoma, with terminal brain cancer becoming a possible unwanted outcome. The time from diagnosis to getting the all-clear was about a month.

There is nothing like the thought of losing your life to elevate your thinking to a whole new level. I started thinking about the things that I am grateful for and things that I would miss.

Leaving Kate and never seeing her again. I just couldn't quite come to grips with this appalling prospect.

I thought about all the incredible experiences that we have had with family and friends. No more milestones for me. Birthdays, weddings, holidays together, hugs, laughs, university capping ceremonies, and so much more, all gone.

And the joy of movement, the daily walks, the scenery, the smell and sound of the sea. The games of golf, tennis, snooker and banter with my mates. No more beer and chips!

I can now totally relate to the inspiring stories that you hear about people who have lived through near-death experiences and survived. In all cases, they have a new heightened zest for life and are immensely grateful for the chance.

In all cases, I'm sure that this gratefulness translates into a new resolution to get the best out of the rest of their lives.

Take some time to write down all of the things that you are grateful for in your life. If you can work on keeping them front of mind, you will inevitably become a much more positive and happier person.

They will also help to shut out much of the negative noise that today's chaotic world throws at us daily.

DIGITAL ISSUES

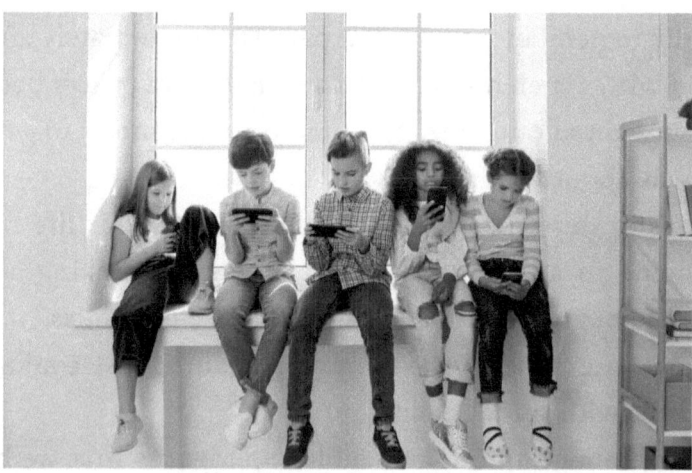

While we are so fortunate to live in this incredibly connected-up world, courtesy of the internet and infinite social media and other platforms, negative aspects also abound. These include long periods of sitting, neck and sight issues, as well as social media and smartphone addictions.

If you are at all unhappy about the relationship you have with all your different devices and platforms, take time out to review this.

DEPRESSION

Although I am definitely not qualified to give advice on this scarily widespread problem, I am aware of some obvious common themes.

If you regularly feel out of sorts mentally and generally unhappy with your life, seek help. Mental health no longer has the stigma attached to it as in the past. It is more mainstream now with lots of avenues for help available. Don't hesitate; talk to your friends and family now about your feelings.

There is no doubt that low mood can become a habit, and you just get used to living your life in a low-quality, fuzzy state.

I can relate to one time in my life where I was probably depressed. This was back in the eighties, after I had become divorced. I thought I was okay and seemed to be muddling along alright.

A couple of years later, my friends put me straight on this. They told me that I had become a right pain. Endlessly asking what I had done to deserve this and painful blow-by-blow analyses of the marital split-up. This was often during or after lengthy boozy sessions at the pub.

I was completely unaware of this at the time, and somehow fortunately came right without medical intervention. Sadly, as we all know, this is often not the case and results in disastrous outcomes.

If you're not right, seek help!

Accept that life is going to throw you many curveballs and you just need to get on and deal with them. Don't 'sweat the small stuff' and spend less time with people that do. And be grateful for all the positive aspects of your life.

MARGARET BORLAND'S STORY

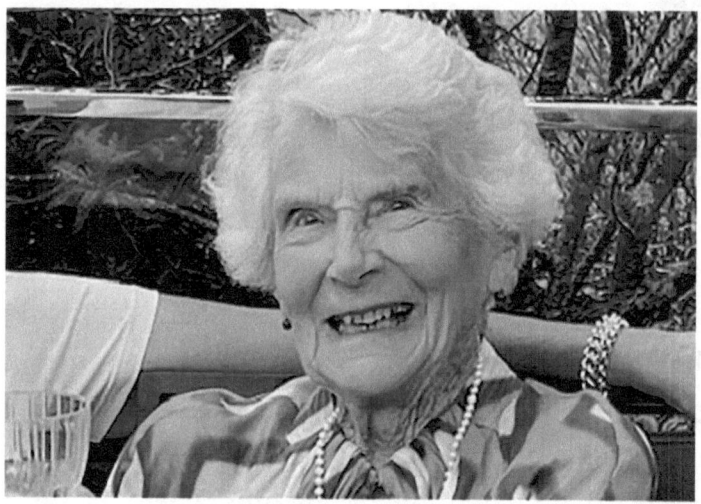

> I was in Dunedin visiting old friends and on hearing that I was writing this book they excitedly told me that I just had to meet their friend Margaret.
>
> And I did. In her ninety-seventh year, Margaret is a remarkably vibrant and fit lady. She is still driving a car, gardening, playing nine-hole golf and bridge and regularly tripping around New Zealand.
>
> I read somewhere recently that women of her generation have a baked-on hard veneer of resilience. Surviving a world war and numerous epidemics over her long life, she totally typifies this description.

Margaret was born as Margaret Pyle in the little town of St Bathans in Central Otago in 1926. This was nearing the end of the gold-mining boom that the town had experienced for many years.

The family owned a farm and the local store. Her grandfather had owned the local store and had grubstaked many of the miners to help in their quest to find gold. Grubstaking was quite common in those early trading days and resulted in goods being swapped for gold.

Only a few years earlier, four of her uncles had fought in the First World War and sadly only two had returned. One of these is portrayed in a display in Te Papa Museum in Wellington as a typical trooper of Gallipoli.

Tragically, her father died in a car accident when Margaret was two years old and she lived the following years alone with her mother.

'I talked to myself a lot and this was mainly to my imaginary friend who was my constant friend over all these years.

'Although this may sound a bit demented, it really did help me to cope with this solitary life.'

The town's school had twenty-one pupils and at age thirteen she was sent to board at Waitaki Girls School in Oamaru.

This was 1939 and Margaret can still remember the day the Second World War started, 'That was a memorable day, and I still remember Prime Minister Michael Savage being on the wireless and hearing through the familiar static, 'Britain is now at war with Germany. Where she goes, we go. Where she stands, we stand.'

Her mother told her that the war wouldn't last long, and soon they were singing patriotically, 'We're going to hang out the washing on the Siegfried Line'.

There was optimism like this at first, which after a while turned into patriotism. This probably toned down the dreadful overall sadness that must have prevailed in this little town.

Margaret vividly recalls 'the boys' being farewelled at the local hall. Harry Sherp was one of these and of German descent. He was also killed in action, and she wondered whether or not he had been fighting men of his own descent.

Julian Tryon came from England and was another name that she remembered. She thought, well, at least he was going back to Europe, close to home. Fortuitously, he survived and came back to farm at the nearby town of Becks.

There were many restrictions and blackouts in Oamaru at night and even an air-raid shelter. 'The stars had never been so bright at night.'

As a precaution the girls were often sent up into the hills with little kits. There was often a fair amount of laughter about all this, and part of their kit was a toilet roll and a wooden clothes peg. The former is obviously practical and the latter was to bite down on when the bombs fell around them. No wonder they used to joke about all this.

From time to time, girls would disappear into the Head's study and reappear in floods of tears. Another dreaded telegram had arrived.

Despite the war, Margaret had five wonderful years at the school before heading off to Dunedin to study physiotherapy at the University of Otago.

One day she and some friends had been riding horses up in Pine Hill. On their return to town all the tram bells were heard clanging, signalling the end of the war. This was VE Day and joyous celebrations broke out in many parts of the world.

She said this was tempered by a deep sadness when they remembered so many of their friends and family who had been killed. The local cinema showed graphic pictures of the ruined cities.

As a newly qualified physiotherapist, Margaret used to enjoy treating the injuries of the returned soldiers. They were positive men, relieved to be home, and apart from their wounds most were in good physical condition.

These were happy and free times and at age twenty-four she married Frank Rennie, a GP with a large practice in South Dunedin. They had three girls, who all became teachers and lived happy and sporty lives in different parts of New Zealand. She noted wryly that they were all pensioners now.

Frank was a sports lover who enjoyed golf, played first-fifteen rugby and was a university blue in cricket.

They enjoyed many happy years together with a constant theme of sport running through their everyday lives. Their travel reflected this and she fondly recalls the 1956 Melbourne Olympics, Wimbledon, a cricket test at Lord's and the 1976 All Blacks rugby tour to South Africa.

'Frank was rugby and cricket mad, and we loved all these occasions. I still remember how simple things were back in the day, particularly the Olympics. I felt dreadful shame in South Africa about apartheid and felt really proud of our Māori players.'

Sadly, her husband Frank passed away at the young age of fifty-six. He had always worked tirelessly in his huge practice, and this had taken its toll on his health.

Coincidentally, I was recently talking to a friend of mine about writing Margaret's story. He remembered that he had gone through Physical Education School in Dunedin with a Rosemary Rennie. Confirming that we do indeed live in a small world, sure enough, this turned out to be one of her daughters.

Margaret has had a lifelong interest in sport going back to her first memories as a young girl playing hockey on the frozen grounds in the Maniototo district. She can still remember the slush and the mud and the frozen fingers and feet. And no surprise that she learned to skate and also the art of curling at a young age.

Her mother had remarried, and her stepfather's curling title was m'lord which was the name of the top man in the district. In 1938 he led a team of twelve curlers to Melbourne to take part in the first ever curling international between the two countries.

Tennis became Margaret's best sport and she always strived to be better than everybody else and used to hit balls against the wall for hours on end.

This competitive attitude resulted in her having a sixty-years-plus tennis career in which she gathered many titles. These included being a nationally ranked singles player, winning a national doubles title, several Otago singles titles and latterly, many masters' titles. She had also been a New Zealand university blue.

She captained two New Zealand masters teams overseas. In the over fifty-five age group she was a winner of an Australasian title.

Apart from her tennis successes, Margaret also became a life member of her local club and the Otago Tennis Association, and a former president of the latter. She says that all this was her other life's work.

All good things come to an end, and at age seventy-six after a knee operation Margaret reluctantly retired from tennis. 'I didn't like not being able to catch up with those drop-shots any more.'

Badminton and golf were her other two favourite games, and she once holed in one at Dunedin's famous Balmacewan course.

After her first husband Frank had passed away, Margaret went back to being a physiotherapist. She remembered the challenges of treating patients during the polio epidemic and also those with tuberculosis.

A number of years later she met Neil Borland who

was the Dean of the Dunedin Teacher's College, and they married and settled in the delightful coastal village of Anderson's Bay just a stone's throw from the city.

Neil had two sons and a daughter, and they both did well to successfully accommodate the needs of each other's family.

One of their special places was Fiordland. Neil introduced Margaret to the wonders of this amazing place, and they walked the beautiful tracks and visited other parts many times.

Neil passed away eleven years ago. Margaret recalls, 'When my first husband died I remember firmly telling myself that I would never let myself be really hurt like this again. After Neil died, I think that this pact I had made with myself all those years ago helped ease the pain.'

Margaret has gradually adapted to her life once again on her own. After sixty-seven years living in (as the locals call it) 'Andy Bay', she is content and loving life in this great environment.

So far we have taken a chronological run through her life which only really scratches the surface. Margaret was born way back in the gold mining era, and here she is nearly a hundred years later amazingly still very hale and hearty. The next and last part of her brilliant life story is to look at how she has managed this.

She tells me that I'm really only a young fellow at

age eighty, as she is seventeen years older. This sounds rather good to me.

I think back seventeen years to when I was sixty-three and still playing pretty full-on tennis singles. Up and down 'The Mount' and playing a round of golf all in the one day and regularly taking on long-distance travel. I realise that seventeen years is a very long time and dread to think what I might be like if I made it to Margaret's age.

I ask her how she stays positive.

'I try to get the most out of things. Sometimes this is hard, but I just don't want to be unhappy even though I know this sounds a bit like Pollyanna.

'It's not to say I'm happy all of the time and sometimes you're desperate.

'My attitude is that I need to always test myself. As a child I always wanted to be somebody and I suppose I still do.

'So I say to myself: c'mon now Margaret. It's a bit like playing a few sets of hard tennis. You just have to keep going.

'Nobody really understands how you feel at this age. They can't because they haven't been here. Although you have support mechanisms, I now have few friends. All my close friends bar two have passed away, and they're not too flash either.'

I ask her how well connected she is to friends and family.

'Well, I am kept so busy. I've just been to lunch with a few of my young golfing seventy-something-year-old friends. They are such fun and we have plenty of laughs.

My book club friends are all graduates and I find their conversations really stimulating. I also play bridge, and this really helps to keep the old brain ticking over.

'It has been too wet for golf today and I expect my gardener to come tomorrow.

'I'm so grateful, not everybody can do all these things.

'I have contact with my daughters and granddaughters on a daily basis. I realise how lucky I am to get so much attention. At the same time, I have a rule that I don't want to become dependent on them.

'If I do have to go into care I will go willingly. In cricketing terms, I will know that I have had an exceptionally good innings.'

She still has her driver's licence and told me a hilarious story about the last time she had to sit this.

'This driving instructor never even asked me my name, just told me to get in. I pigheadedly asked him what his qualifications were for the job, and instantly recognised that this was probably the wrong question to ask.

'I was right, and long story short he failed me. It was something to do with driving too slowly through intersections. I thought this should have been a good thing.

'On booking for a re-test, I asked within his hearing what choice of instructor I had. "None" was the answer, and I thought that this might have been my second mistake of the day. Third that is; I had forgotten about the intersection problem.

'Thankfully, this was not to be, as after having some driving lessons I came back and passed after being tested by the same man.

'So, you see, never give up!'

I ask Margaret about her general health. She feels really good about her health and surmises that is because she is still in good health.

This is with one reservation and the fly in the ointment. She has been recently diagnosed with macular degeneration and takes pills and visits the clinic once a month.

She loves her reading and is finding this a bit more difficult as she feels something lurking there in her eyes.

She repeats again that she is very grateful for her long and healthy life. She worries about the many people that don't have much and concludes that many make do and are happy despite this.

Although not a fanatic, Margaret walks every day and knows her limitations. She enjoys the hills and also has a steep path in her garden. Her friends tell her that this and the stairs in her house are dangerous. She disagrees and says that they help to keep her fit.

I agree. She does, however, cut herself a bit of slack.

'I now play my golf at Chisholm Park links which is closer to home and much flatter than Balmacewan.

'I'm not all that marvellous either you know. My gardener even found me asleep on my sofa the other day. And recently I got overenthusiastic in the hills and strained my Achilles tendon.

'I have this huge mirror at the top of my stairs. One day I thought I looked particularly gorgeous and after giving myself a big smile collapsed in a heap. This is my only big fall, and I recovered quite quickly from this.

'I also broke my big toe and received no sympathy at all.

'I move really quickly in the garden, and I am quite worried that I will have a fall out there one day.'

She receives Meals on Wheels three times a week and uses these to supplement the fruit and veg she harvests from her garden. She is not too big on meat and gets her protein from other sources like fish, cheese and other dairy products.

She enjoys a drink most nights and admits to a couple of glasses of wine sometimes.

Margaret says, 'I grew up in a drink culture and remember a childhood swamped in whisky. I didn't like it much. Despite this I enjoy a drink most nights and enjoy a get-together with my girls over a drink or two.'

I ask her about her weight and, unsurprisingly for one so active, she's a size eight at 1.60 metres tall (five feet three inches) and weighing just over fifty kilograms (eight stone). As a younger woman, she was a size twelve and few kilograms heavier.

One of her daughters told her the other day that her shoulder blades stuck out so much they looked like wings. Family are good like that.

On that note we ended our talk and what a pleasure and a privilege this was.

In searching for one word that would describe Margaret, I came up with 'irrepressible'. After all the ups and downs and hurly-burly of a long and active life, she still somehow is full of humour, optimism and energy.

While genetics certainly play a part in what any individual's healthspan years may be, everything that I have read and experienced points to about 80 per cent of this coming down to attitude.

Margaret obviously has a great attitude to life. She is fit and active, socially well-connected, a healthy weight, regularly challenges herself and certainly has purpose to her life.

A wonderful sense of humour and a tenacious spirit are also both great assets in coping with the inevitable demands of living well into one's nineties and beyond. This sounds like a real privilege, and at the same time a great challenge. Margaret is well equipped to accept and enjoy both criteria.

5

HORMONES, METABOLIC SYNDROME AND DIETARY SUPPLEMENTS

KEY POINTS

- **Hormones** are known as the body's chemical messengers. They carry signals from glands through the bloodstream to tissues and organs.
- **Metabolic Syndrome** is the name for a group of factors which significantly increase your risk of stroke, heart attack and other health problems. They include a large waist, high blood pressure and high blood sugar levels.
- **Dietary supplements** are taken to provide a positive adjustment to an area of the body where there might be a deficiency.
- **Electrolytes** – A GP may include screening of electrolytes when you have a blood test. Electrolytes are chemicals in your blood like zinc, sodium, iron, calcium, magnesium,

potassium and phosphates. If they are outside the normal range, your GP will suggest a course of action.
- **Vitamins** – Vitamins A, B, C, D, E, B12 and others are essential parts of a healthy diet and can be found in a wide variety of foods.

In this chapter we look at three important areas of your health which are either often misunderstood or quite simply not even on your radar.

HORMONES

Hormones are known as the body's chemical messengers. They are powerful agents and are of great importance. They carry signals from glands through the bloodstream to tissues and organs.

Insulin

Before 1921, type 1 diabetics would die shortly after their condition was diagnosed. Frederick Banting, a Canadian surgeon working in the University of Toronto, discovered that insulin, which was made by the pancreas, could be sourced from outside the human body. Initial animal sources for insulin were dogs, calves and then cattle and pigs. Today, insulin is made by genetic engineering.

In 1922, Leonard Thompson, a fourteen-year-old boy dying from type 1 diabetes, was successfully treated with an injection of insulin. There was much joy and celebration, and a Nobel Prize followed for Banting and the two scientists who worked with him.

Insulin helps to move glucose from the bloodstream into your cells. Diabetics have too much glucose in their bloodstream and their pancreas cannot keep up with enough supply to correct this.

The excess glucose lays down plaque which narrows blood vessels and can cause stroke, heart disease, amputations, kidney failure and other life-threatening conditions.

Injected insulin helps to restore blood sugar levels to normal. Research towards an insulin pill is advancing.

Type 1 diabetics have a pancreas which makes no insulin or not enough to have normal blood sugar levels.

The majority of cases of type 2 diabetes are caused by people's lifestyle choices and can often be remedied by the right dietary interventions.

Thyroxine

The thyroid gland is in your neck and makes the hormone thyroxine. Thyroxine helps to control your growth and development.

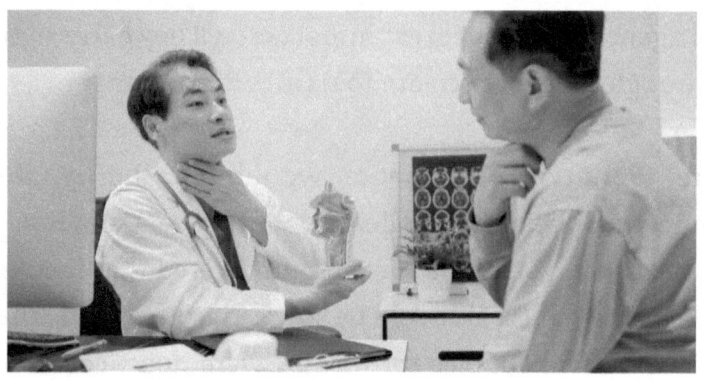

Too little thyroxine will slow your metabolic rate. This is called hypothyroidism and also slows down the rate you can burn energy (calories). You're likely to put on weight and other symptoms are hair loss and feeling cold and generally fatigued.

Fortunately, synthetic thyroxine can be prescribed by your doctor to speed things up.

Too much thyroxine causes a condition called hyperthyroidism and symptoms include anxiety, hyperactivity, heat sensitivity and fatigue.

The thyroid stimulating hormone (TSH) is released by the brain to stimulate thyroxine production and a simple blood test can check that your levels are okay. The higher your TSH levels, the lower your thyroid activity.

There seem to be two schools of thought on what the normal range should be. It is often said that between 0.3 and 5.0 is normal, although other experts like to see the level no higher than 3.0.

The stress hormones: adrenaline and cortisol

These hormones are made by your adrenal glands, which sit above your kidneys.

Adrenaline is your 'fight or flight' hormone and is quickly released in times of high stress, like being in imminent danger.

We all know or have heard stories about miraculous shows of strength. Lifting a car off a trapped person or jumping a high fence to avoid a charging bull are two that come to mind.

Adrenaline can certainly be your friend. However, one of the effects of adrenaline is to raise blood sugar levels (very useful for fighting or fleeing). A stressful life, particularly if it is fairly sedentary, can result in adrenaline, causing blood sugar spikes. Prolonged and frequent periods of high blood sugar can lead to weight and diabetes issues.

Cortisol can also be your friend or foe. The right amount reduces inflammation and helps control insulin production.

Too much continual stress causes high cortisol levels. This results in raised blood sugar levels, higher insulin demand and results in weight gain.

. . .

Sex hormones

Once again these are powerful agents and crucial to a happy and healthy life. The two main ones for females are **oestrogen and progesterone** and the right balance between the two is essential.

The former helps to shape the curves of the body. Excess oestrogen will help to lay down fat in the wrong places and leads to a pear-shaped appearance. It can also cause fluid retention, headaches and a low libido.

Progesterone is charged with helping with conception and has antidepressant and diuretic benefits.

Getting the balance right is essential. Oestrogen dominance can cause many problems which include weight gain, migraines, painful periods and mood swings.

A blood test will establish what your own levels are. Your doctor will refer you to a specialist if required.

Testosterone is mainly a male hormone and helps develop reproductive tissues, promote bone and muscle growth, and is essential for overall health. Low testosterone levels are common in males as they age, and large waistlines and low libido are common outcomes.

Last year an old cricketing friend of mine told me that he was exhibiting both of the above symptoms. A blood test revealed low testosterone levels. The application of skin patches and a gel eventually resulted in a much happier and lighter old mate.

METABOLIC SYNDROME

This is the name for a group of factors which significantly increase your risk of stroke, heart attack and other health problems.

Factors include:

- A large waist – fat in this area carries a greater risk than fat in other parts of the body
- High blood pressure
- High triglycerides – this is having too much fat in your blood
- High blood sugar levels
- Cholesterol abnormalities

This syndrome is closely linked to the obesity and diabetes epidemics. If you have these sorts of issues, you will also find it difficult to lose weight.

Your doctor will suggest a blood test and will routinely take your blood pressure and your waist measurement. If you think you may be heading in this direction, pay immediate attention and do something about it.

DIETARY SUPPLEMENTS

Dietary supplements are taken to provide a positive adjustment to an area of the body where there might be a deficiency.

The supplement market worldwide is massive and catering to what seems an insatiable demand. No doubt accompanying this trend is a fair amount of wasted dollars. This would either be on products that are not up to the job or others which are simply not targeted at the right need.

I am only going to cover a few supplements I am familiar with and where I am confident of their importance if there is a deficiency in this area.

The efficacy of particular product choices is tricky. My rule of thumb is twofold. Check out independent comments on the supplements, particularly from well-qualified health professionals.

Do not rely entirely on product suppliers' endorsements even if they are from one of your favourite film stars.

Also, if possible go for supplements that have met some industry standards or scientific analysis. Better still if they have been developed by doctors and scientists and rigorously tested.

Magnesium (Mg)

This is my first cab off the rank because of the importance and effectiveness of this trace element supplement.

Foods rich in magnesium include leafy greens, avocado, fish, nuts, seeds and beans.

Magnesium is found throughout the body and is the subject of many scientific studies whose findings include the following benefits:

- Acts as a helper molecule in many biochemical reactions including converting food into energy, formation of protein, muscle movement and nervous system regulation
- Combatting depression
- Maintaining normal blood sugar levels
- Anti-inflammatory properties
- Bone and heart health

I used to suffer from quite severe regular cramping in both the calf and hamstring areas. At times I could actually see the calf muscles twitching. After having taken magnesium supplements for some time now, these regular symptoms have almost disappeared.

On the advice of a naturopath, I take magnesium citrate capsules as they are easier on your gut than their magnesium oxide equivalents.

For the odd night-time cramping event I take one or two dissolvable magnesium phosphate tissue salts which I put under my tongue. They seem to work quite quickly and effectively.

I also know people who swear by magnesium supplements in helping them to sleep better.

Some symptoms of magnesium deficiency include nausea, fatigue, pins and needles, hyperexcitability and loss of appetite. A number of scientific studies indicate that up to half of those studied were magnesium deficient.

If you exhibit any of these symptoms, you could try magnesium citrate capsules to see if there is any improvement.

Glucosamine and chondroitin

This combo supplement is said to help with the mobility, lubrication and cushioning of joints.

Many years ago, I bought a big tub of these to help with joint pain that I had in my hips and ankles. After taking two capsules a day for a few months I certainly noticed a difference.

The big tub eventually ran out. I didn't replace it and a few months later these symptoms reappeared. I purchased another big tub and have used this supplement successfully ever since.

A friend of mine used to have a flighty, patchwork-patterned mongrel that over the years had become quite arthritic and slow-moving.

Much to my surprise, after being away for about a year, this same dog Benji bounded out of their driveway to greet me. Turns out that my old friend Dick had been taking these same joint supplements and decided to try them out on Benji. He crushed them up to put with his food, and a couple of months later was amazed when the dog's mobility started to improve.

Scientific studies provide mixed results on this supplement's efficacy for the treatment of osteoarthritis. On the other hand, studies have proved that this supplement has anti-inflammatory properties which help reduce pain in joints.

This supplement mix has worked for both me and the dog. If you have joint issues, my advice would be to give this supplement mix a go. It will take two or more months for you to notice any difference in pain levels. In my case, in line with the studies, the key benefit was in the reduction in pain.

VITAMIN D

This vitamin is produced in our skin and sunlight is vital in its production. *Among other benefits it is critical for building bones, boosting immunity and reducing inflammation.*

Studies have shown epidemic numbers of people around the world are vitamin D deficient. A deficiency of vitamin D presents with similar symptoms to those from a lack of magnesium.

Fortunately, the remedies for this are simple. It is often due to a lack of sunshine. The late afternoon is best to safely increase your exposure to the sun for short periods.

If a blood test indicates low vitamin D levels, your GP will prescribe vitamin D3 supplements. The prescribed version is a high-dose supplement and far more effective than over-the-counter counterparts.

ELECTROLYTES

A GP may include screening of electrolytes when you have a blood test. Electrolytes are chemicals in your blood like zinc, sodium, iron, calcium, magnesium, potassium and phosphates.

If they are outside the normal range, your GP will suggest a course of action. For example, it could be that you have low sodium levels. You will either not be having enough sodium in your diet or you could be drinking too much water.

The latter is definitely a thing, not too uncommon, and can cause the leaching out of sodium and other electrolytes.

A few years ago, I started suffering from nausea and became quite fatigued. Low sodium levels were diagnosed, and I started monitoring and reducing my water intake. Within a week or two, my symptoms disappeared and a blood test revealed normal levels again.

As with low magnesium levels, you can experience a similar range of symptoms which make you feel unwell. A blood test can sort out what's wrong and a course of action put in place. This may take a bit of juggling to get right.

There are specific supplements like iron, calcium and magnesium that you can take which make sense if one of these is shown to be deficient.

OTHER VITAMINS

Vitamins A, B, C, D, E, B12 and others are essential parts of a healthy diet and can be found in a wide variety of foods.

If you are still feeling unwell despite all of your blood test results being normal, a vitamin deficiency could be the problem. Although one or two of these are expensive, like the vitamin D test, there are individual blood tests available for most vitamins.

The jury seems to be out on the effectiveness of taking a regular multivitamin supplement. Nonetheless, this is a multibillion-dollar industry, and although you can get sufficient vitamins and minerals from a varied diet, I would not rule out taking a high-quality multivitamin supplement.

BLOOD TEST

If you ever feel unwell over an extended period with symptoms like nausea, fatigue, headaches or muscle cramps, a blood test is a must. Your doctor will organise the relevant tests for you.

6

DEALING WITH INJURIES AND OTHER ACHES AND PAINS

KEY POINTS

- **Basic principles** – It helps to have a clear view of what to do when you get injured. For example, with a soft tissue injury, first apply the RICE method and follow this up with an x-ray and/or ultrasound if necessary.
- **Do the hard yards on rehab** – Some of the treatment can be painful and it is crucial not to shirk on this and continue the stretches and other exercises well after the symptoms have gone away.
- **Beware atrophy** – Muscles will begin to waste very quickly after an injury and will lose strength and size. It is vital to get back to normal movement as soon as possible to keep this to a minimum.
- **Second opinion** – If you are not happy with your diagnosis or treatment for any injury or other problem,

seek a second opinion. Do not let long periods drag on with no apparent improvement.
- **Posture and gait** – After an injury it is natural to favour the affected area. This can often lead to a change in your gait. Your posture can also be compromised. Shoulders back, stand square and tall and don't forget to check out your gait.
- **Love those tennis balls** – These are great to roll around various parts of your body to relieve tension and pain.
- **Know the nature of the beast** – If you can learn a little basic anatomy, this can help motivate you when you are trying to recover from injury.
- **Movement is your biggest asset** – Take every opportunity that you reasonably have to move and stretch. Always break up long periods of sitting with some form of movement.

I played a number of sports competitively for a long period of time and taught Physical Education until I was forty years old.

Inevitably, this has led to more than a few mishaps. This chapter is about what I have learned from these wide-ranging experiences. Some of these insights have helped me immeasurably to stay up and running.

TYPES OF INJURIES

There are basically two types of injuries, bone and soft tissues. The former is self-explanatory, and the latter involves the soft tissues of the body including muscles, tendons, ligaments, cartilages and nerves. I will concentrate far more on soft-tissue injuries.

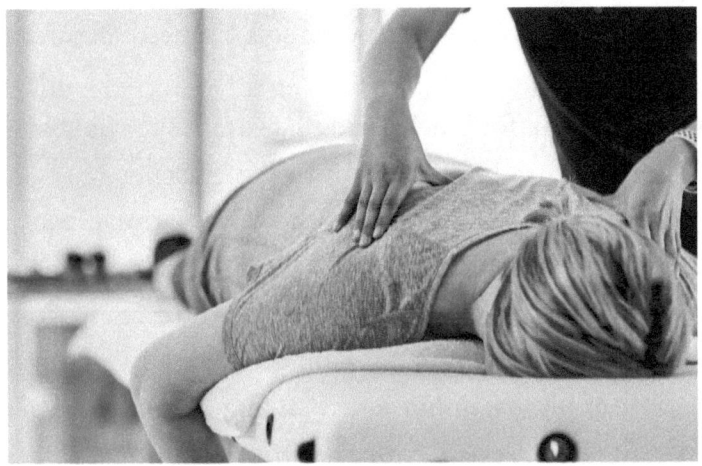

The reason is that if you do have an accident and think that you have broken or fractured a bone, your first course of action is to get it x-rayed. The result of your x-ray will dictate what treatment will follow. Serious injuries resulting in a number of broken bones and soft-tissue injuries often will require surgery and ongoing treatment. Often with a simple fracture or break, you will simply need to commit to time in a plaster cast or moon boot.

On the other hand, the diagnosis and treatments for soft-tissue injuries are wide-ranging and sometimes complex. Ankle injuries are a good example. My recovery from an ankle injury has many elements common to other soft-tissue injuries. Back in my mid-thirties in my teaching days, after going up for a block during a game of volleyball, I landed on someone's foot and twisted my ankle badly. Apart from the embarrassment of crashing to the ground with all the kids crowding around, the pain was immense and I can remember my foot shaking uncontrollably.

At the hospital, the bone x-ray was all clear. The diagnosis was a badly sprained ankle with considerable swelling and some damage done to tendons, ligaments and other soft tissues. Fortunately, none of these required surgery.

I was strapped up for weeks and on crutches for part of this time. An ultrasound was used to check out the soft tissues.

In the initial stages I followed the RICE principle of rest, ice, compression and elevation.

After a few days and once the swelling had come down, I was back on my feet again trying to walk as normally as possible. *This was a key part of my rehabilitation. Walking around helped to get the circulation going and prevent atrophy of the leg muscles. This wasting of muscle can occur quite quickly and should be avoided if possible.*

Anyone who has had a limb in a plaster cast for some time will attest to this. It is incredible how much smaller and weaker the limb can become. And getting the muscles and other tissues back to normal is quite a mission.

I always tend to err on the side of getting up and running as quickly as possible. In this case, with the ankle still strapped up and taking regular Panadol, I was happy to put up with some minor pain to be able to get walking without crutches again.

During PE classes I would ask a couple of the kids to tell me how even my gait was when I was walking or running around. They would often say that I looked a bit lopsided.

It is a common occurrence after a serious ankle or leg injury to still favour the injured bit. It is vital to be aware of this and to try to work on having a symmetrical gait, otherwise a permanent limp can result. Sometimes, in more serious cases this cannot be avoided.

An important part of the rehabilitation was time spent on a wobble board and doing various stretching exercises. A wobble board is a round board with a half-ball of wood attached to the bottom of it. It is big enough for you to stand on with both feet, and believe me you wobble around alright. It is a great bit of gear and helped with my balance and the strengthening of my ankle.

My physio was old-school and she really got stuck in with 'diggy' fingers into the tendons that had some adhesions on the bony inner part of my ankle.

Oh my goodness, what a painful process that was, and it made me break out in a real sweat. I realised that it was for my own good and gritted my teeth accordingly.

I wish that I had had that sort of fortitude in my earlier years. At a fairly torrid university party I had an accident with a Bowie knife which ended up with me slicing both sets of flexor tendons in each of the last three fingers of my right hand. These are the ones that help you to make a fist. Although my memory of this night is a bit hazy, I can remember half the party trooping down to Casualty with me. They would have got short shrift, and I was stitched up and sent home to sober up.

The next day I went back, and in a four-hour op they were able to fish around to find the separated tendons and stitch them together. Unfortunately, they were set in fixed flexion which meant they were not quite straight. After the plaster came off, I was sent to the local hospital for physio.

Now this part I do remember. In walked a fearsome-looking giant of a woman. Her two weapons of choice were a hot wax bath and a metal dish full of ice. This was the old hot and cold treatment.

What followed was an hour of horror. She pummelled my fingers for about half of this trying to straighten them and then proceeded to instruct me to plunge my hand alternately into the hot wax and then into the ice dish.

Quite idiotically, I never returned for another round of this treatment. These three fingers remain slightly flexed to this day.

Perhaps if I had persevered, they might have come right. I'll never know.

Some rehab steps

My insights from the ankle injury are simple: As soon as possible apply the *RICE principles – rest, ice, compression and elevation. To avoid muscle wasting, stay positive, get back walking as soon as reasonably possible and do the hard yards on rehab.*

Adhesions are fibrous tissues which attach to tendons and other soft tissues as our body's response to injury and overuse. They actually feel like little knots and can cause pain and weaken and cause stiffness in that area.

If adhesions occur, you can help resolve these by running a tennis ball or similar over them for a few minutes or using your own 'diggy' fingers. Be firm with both methods and you should feel some pain without it being severe. You can repeat this regularly for a few minutes at a time.

If the problem persists, go back to your physio for further treatment.

'Diggy' fingers and other types of massage help to improve both blood and lymph flow, relieve tension in muscles and reduce pain.

Your gait – Make sure your gait is even. Staying symmetrical is vital to avoid any permanent limping and potentially other problems down the track.

NORDIC WALKING

This is walking using two special poles, one in each hand. Each time you take a step forward with your right foot the end of the pole in your left hand is placed on the ground in front of you for leverage and balance. You repeat this routine with your other leg.

Although this may sound complicated, it comes quite naturally as it mirrors the exact sequence you are using with your legs stepping and your arms swinging.

I am a big fan of this walking for a number of reasons, and scientific studies back up the following benefits. Two of my friends who are struggling with their mobility, on trying these poles out immediately had more confidence and stability in their walking action and the length of their step.

Nordic walking can result in increased cardiovascular benefits compared with regular walking, improved balance and stability, upper body muscle development, positive effects for older adults and potential for rehabilitation.

My primary interest is in helping older people who are walking with a stick and who have some strength and balance issues.

I remember a close friend of mine with Parkinson's walking with a stick and becoming quite tipped over towards the side the stick was on. I suggested that she use a walker and immediately she became more balanced and symmetrical, and her confidence improved dramatically.

Perhaps she could have taken the step up to using the Nordic poles and improved even more. I never thought of this at the time, and she now has moved to another part of the country.

I think there is enormous potential for rehabilitation using these poles and keen to follow up on this and continue to support my two friends who have just started to use these brilliant walking aids.

TENNIS BALLS

Tennis balls are not just for playing tennis – I have found that they are my go-to bit of gear for many injuries that I have had.

Although quite pliable, they can still give different areas of the body a workout when applied with some force. And, of course, you can roll around on them.

With my ankle injury, I roll a tennis ball under my foot to help relieve tension in the tendons. I tend to concentrate on the area near the highest part of the arch and put on as much pressure as I can for about two minutes.

With both hands, I also roll a ball up and down my calf muscles with as much force as I can for about thirty seconds at a time. This is also to relieve tension in these muscles and tendons.

UNDERSTANDING ANATOMY

With any particular problem that we face it always helps to have a good understanding of all of the factors involved.

Although my ankle injury occurred over forty-years ago, I still periodically have problems with it. This often results in pain around my heel and the inside of the ankle.

My physio has shown me diagrams of the anatomy in this area and explained why I get pain here. This really helps me to stay motivated over the period it takes to put things right.

Just below the round bony bit that sticks out on the inside of your ankle above your heel run nerves, an artery and tendons. These flexor tendons insert on your big toe and run all the way back up your calf to their origin at the top of the knee.

These powerful flexor muscles are located deep in our calves. They help us to flex our big toe and stand on our tiptoes. If the tendons get shortened or damaged in some way, it will cause tension and pain in busy areas like this one I have mentioned above.

Now that I understand this, I am far happier doing both the

painful 'diggy' fingers exercises on my ankle and foam roller ones on my calves to help repair and lengthen these tendons.

When you visit your physio, if one is not offered, always ask for an explanation about the nature of your injury.

SOME COMMON AILMENTS

Lower back

A common area for problems is the lower back. When I finished teaching in 1984 my lumbar sacral area was as stiff as a board. Instead of having a nice little curve, it was completely straight and unyielding.

Even as a physical education teacher always talking about the benefits of stretching, I had somehow neglected this key area of my body.

The vertebrae, muscles and other soft tissues in this area all need to move easily together during movement. Imagine me landing after, say, doing a jump in volleyball. Instead of a nice cushioning effect, I was getting a good old jarring as there was quite simply no give.

I had continual pain in this area and many people experience the same thing. Pain killers and anti-inflammatories will only mask the symptoms.

Two key stretches – It was quite a mission to re-educate this long-neglected area. I used two key stretches which I have covered earlier but will set out again below in more detail. The trick is to both loosen up the structures in this area and restore the gentle spinal curve.

Knees up – The first exercise is to lie on your back with your legs out straight. Bring one knee up and with both hands draw it upwards as far as you can towards your chest. Hold for fifteen seconds and repeat with the other leg.

I also do this same exercise standing. This comes in handy when you are out and about and feel your back stiffening up.

Buttock rolls – The second exercise is also done on your back with knees bent and feet on the floor. Have both elbows and the palms of your hands on the ground.

Gently roll your buttocks in the direction of your feet. You will feel your back arch in your lower back region. Hold briefly, before pushing your buttocks along the ground back towards your head. You should feel the arch in your lower back straighten and almost push down into the ground.

You can also do this exercise standing and effectively use gravity to give you a bit more push.

Stand with your back to the wall with feet apart and heels a few centimetres away from the wall. Leaving your buttocks in the same place, slightly bend you knees till you feel the lower back arch. Hold briefly, before straightening your legs and going up slightly onto your toes to help push the middle of your lower back into the wall.

It took me a couple of months before I could feel my lower back arch and some flexibility returning.

From a standing position I also used to turn my trunk around from side to side a few times to help loosen up this area. A wheat-bag also came in handy from time to time.

Ideally you should do sets of these exercises each day. Sets of ten are about right. I still do these same exercises several times a day to retain flexibility in this key area.

Lower back pain can be debilitating and seems to affect almost every movement that you make and is painful even when you are at rest.

These exercises are only effective if you commit to a regime of several sets a day. Once you have flexibility restored, continue the exercises on a regular basis.

Be patient; it took me a long time to see an improvement in this tricky area. If you are not seeing any improvement, book a session with a physio to get you on the right track.

The pelvic region

This is a complex and crowded area. Although I will only cover my own experience with injuries, similar diagnostic and treatment practices will apply for other areas.

Anywhere in the body you can get referred pain. This means that the pain occurs above or below where the real problem is located. I had pain occurring in both my medial gluteal muscle and my groin. The medial glute is a large muscle that helps to stabilise your pelvis and keep you upright when walking and running. Put your hands on your hips on about your belt line and slide your thumbs down a centimetre or two. This is the top of the medial glute and it runs down to insert around the bony bit that sticks out at the top of your hip.

As with all soft-tissue injuries that I can't deal with myself, I started with an appointment with my physio. She massaged this area with the view to freeing up the adhesions in the glute muscle. A set of exercises were agreed on.

My go-to stretch for this area as it isolates this medial glute is as follows. I sit on the very edge of a chair and put my left ankle on top of my right knee. Keeping my back straight, I lean forward until I feel the stretch in the muscle. I hold for about fifteen-seconds and add pressure as I see fit. Repeat with the other leg and do at least three sets of this.

There are other exercises to stretch and strengthen this large muscle which you can find via Google.

After about a week, both the referred pain in my groin and the muscle pain and stiffness improved markedly. I still do this exercise daily to keep this area supple and pain free.

Tennis ball rolling – I lie on my back with knees bent and elbows and palms of my hand on the ground beside my hips.

I put a ball in the middle of the medial glute on each side and roll around on these until they find the sore spots in the muscle. In my case, on the right side there is a very gristly area which kind of has a grinding feeling as I massage this tender spot. This definitely helps relieve pain and loosen things up.

Pelvic floor pain

The pelvic floor area is a crowded and complex area in both men and women. In my case back a few years ago I experienced penile, testicle and other general pelvic floor pain.

After much prodding and poking, blood tests, an MRI and a prostate ultrasound, the diagnosis was benign prostatic hyperplasia (BPH). As men age, this is a common condition which causes the prostate to enlarge. This can cause restricted urine flow and result in a higher frequency of urination. There are a number of options for treatment, and one of these oddly is an injection of Botox. In my case a small dose of a drug called doxazosin thankfully did the trick in helping to improve my urine flow.

It did not help my ongoing pain which, although not confirmed, was thought to be caused by an entrapment of the pudendal nerve which runs through the pelvic floor.

From day one I always thought this was neuromuscular pain, and some of my medical contacts agreed with this. Unfortunately, this was not enough to convince the doctors at a medical practice that I had recently joined.

This resulted in about three months of continuous pain and sleepless nights. Drugs like morphine and sleeping tablets were prescribed. Although the latter were useful in helping me to sleep, the morphine did not help with the pain.

I finally was able to get into a pain specialist who immediately prescribed gabapentin and advised me to gradually wind this up to the maximum dose. The maximum dose was twelve 300- milligram tablets a day for a whopping total of 3600 milligrams. I'm only a fairly little guy and at times I could feel my brain buzzing away and this created a sort of a strange chemical haze. After a short period of time the pain started to recede and I was soon back to normal. What a relief this was and with no noticeable side-effects.

This once again backs up the important idea of continuing to speak up if you are not happy with the treatment that you are getting for any medical condition.

Most health professionals will admit, or should I say should admit, that their diagnosis may not always be right. And, if you are not happy, get a second opinion.

Levator ani syndrome

Levator ani is a muscle group on either side of the pelvis and comprises the main pelvic floor muscle. Levator ani syndrome is episodic rectal pain caused by spasm of the levator ani muscle. This is a painful condition that I get periodically. I use hamstring stretches and sit on tennis balls to help alleviate the pain.

Originally, I had this condition diagnosed as haemorrhoids and was prescribed pile cream. I soon discovered that this did not work. Eventually, a physio successfully diagnosed this condition as levator ani syndrome and agreed with the exercises that I was doing.

Some physios specialise in internal massage inside your anal canal to relieve tension in the muscles. I have had a couple of sessions of this, and although it felt a bit weird, seemed to achieve what it set out to do.

Pelvic floor pain in both men and women is very common and the cause of the pain is often difficult to diagnose. The list of possibilities is enormous and includes urinary tract infections, muscle tension, menstrual pain, endometriosis, nerve pain, haemorrhoids and prostatitis to name a few.

A Headache in the Pelvis is a book written by David Wise and Robert Anderson offers a new visionary approach to problems in the pelvic region. These new methods were developed at Stanford University.

I have read this book and would recommend it to anyone who is experiencing pain in this area and more particularly if a diagnosis is proving to be difficult. It certainly gave me some great insights, and I still use a couple of their ideas.

Head and neck

The weight of an average head is five kilograms (about eleven pounds). This weight sits upon the seven vertebrae in the cervical spine and is supported by twenty muscles. These muscles help the head and neck to move around and keep the head in place.

If we bend our head and neck to a thirty-degree angle forward, this creates a force of eighteen kilos (forty pounds) on our cervical spine. No wonder our neck and upper spine take a hammering with all the various head turns and other movements we expect from it each day.

Stiff and sore necks and shoulders are very commonplace, and 'Text Neck' is definitely now a thing. Imagine the strain on your head and neck that occurs from long periods of texting or checking your social media on your phone. Something's got to give, and it does.

A group of four exercises – I use the combination of exercises already described in the chapter on 'Physical Foundation Blocks'.

They are triceps stretches followed by backward shoulder rolls, head turning from side to side and circular rolling movements of the head and neck.

I use this combination two or three times daily when I feel any stiffness or tension in my neck.

Thumb pain

I regularly experienced pain and stiffness in my right thumb. After many years of tennis, golf, cricket and other sports, this is not surprising.

On having the thumb area x-rayed I found that there was some arthritis. I was told that pain can be alleviated by regularly mobilising the area. I googled this and found two exercises that I could do and one pressure-point.

Holding my hands down by my sides, I alternately flex my wrist up and down followed by rotating my wrist backwards and forwards for about a minute. I do these movements quickly.

This pressure point is found in the space at the base of the thumb and the forefinger. It is called pressure point LI-4. If I continue to have pain in my thumb, I press on this area with my other thumb for about thirty seconds.

I have found that this combination of exercises, which effectively mobilise the thumb well, and the use of the pressure point, have improved the pain that I formerly had quite markedly.

7
LOWERING YOUR BIOLOGICAL AGE

KEY POINTS

- You can form new lifestyle habits which will add years of healthy life.
- With this simple and practical approach Eat For Keeps helped thousands of people with weight and diabetes issues. With a few tweaks I am now applying this same approach to my new programme, The Don't Act Your Age Challenge.
- Your chronological age is based on how many years you have been alive; your biological age is the true age that your cells, tissues and organ systems appear to be, based on biochemistry.
- Epigenetics is the study of the environment you live in and how you behave in it. Your behaviours and environment can cause changes that affect the way your

- genes work. Unlike genetic changes (mutations), epigenetic changes are reversible.
- Over the past decade or so there have been several methods for working out your biological age.
- If you live in a stressful environment, have a stressful job, eat all the wrong types of food and lead a sedentary lifestyle, your mind and body will suffer accordingly.
- Although your DNA will not change, you will not be sending out the right signals to your genes and your biochemistry will suffer accordingly.
- If you lead a relatively stress-free life, eat well and exercise regularly, your rate of ageing is likely to be quite low and you will remain young well into your old age.
- About 80 per cent of your future health will depend on your environment and how you behave in it. Only about 20 per cent is related to your inherited DNA and genes.
- Eating well, hydrating regularly, keeping your body moving and living a relatively stress-free life are some of the basics you need to be aware of.

FORMING NEW HABITS

The *Oxford Dictionary*'s definition of 'method' is 'The quality of being well organised and systematic in thought or action'. My primary objective is to apply this same quality to help people to form new lifestyle habits which will add to their years of healthy life.

My methodical approach to achieve these sometimes life-changing new habits has been developed from my experiences both as a life coach and with the Eat For Keeps programme.

As a life coach, we were trained to provide clarity by keeping any information given to clients as specific and succinct as possible. We encouraged clients to find their own solutions to the various challenges that they would face and to make a few permanent changes to their food choices and lifestyle. This simple and practical approach helped thousands of people with weight and diabetes issues.

With a few tweaks I am now applying this same approach to my new programme, The Don't Act Your Age Challenge.

Having read my book so far you will have possibly made a few lifestyle changes. These are all good steps in the right direction. The hardest part now is having the awareness and motivation to keep these good habits going and even building on them.

Well, the good news is that I have saved the best bit till last and hopefully this will provide you with the ultimate motivation to keep going.

BIOLOGICAL VS CHRONOLOGICAL AGE

While I have discussed this concept of biological age already, it is time now to show you just how life-changing making the right lifestyle changes can be.

Your chronological age is the number of years you have been alive; your biological age is the true age that your cells, tissues and organ systems appear to be, based on biochemistry.

By reversing some of the damage done to your trillions of cells you will become biologically younger.

You can achieve this by taking on The Don't Act Your Age Challenge, which is detailed in the next and final chapter of this book. It is about helping you to form new lifestyle habits which will add to your years of healthy life.

EPIGENETICS

The first step is to take you back through a short history of this natural phenomenon and the study of epigenetics.

Epigenetics is the study of the environment you live in and how you behave in it. Your behaviours and environment can cause changes that affect the way your genes work. Unlike genetic changes (mutations), however, epigenetic changes can be reversed.

Your DNA is responsible for building and maintaining all of your body's structures. Genes are the part of your DNA which gives you the characteristics that make you unique. They work together to provide instructions that tell your cells how to behave. Genomes are groups of genes.

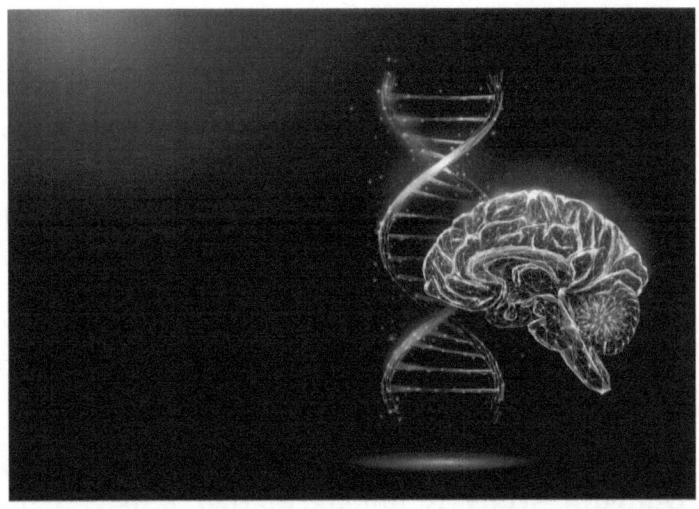

Telomeres are the ends of the DNA molecules and are like the aglets, the little cylindrical things which protect the ends of your shoelaces. When these aglets get damaged, the ends of our shoelaces can become frayed. And likewise, as we age our telomeres become shortened, making damage to your DNA more likely.

Epigenomes are chemical compounds that tell groups of genes what to do, when to do it and where to do it. All going well, these epigenomes and subsequently the genes get all their messages and actions right and all of your body's processes continue to work in sync.

Any damage to your DNA, telomeres or epigenomes can mean that you can get the wrong messages and instead of a set of genes being turned off they remain turned on, or vice versa.

This departure from the norm can cause changes to your cells which can potentially result in a number of medical conditions, ranging from major malformations through to autism and some cancers.

Calculating biological age

Over the past decade or so there have been several methods for working out your biological age developed. 'Epigenetic clocks' use what's called DNA methylation to achieve this.

Back in the early 1970s a new study began in Dunedin, New Zealand. This unique longitudinal study began with 1037 participants all born between 1972 and 1973. Participants have had measures like their lifestyle choices, weight, height, blood-pressure, hormones, cholesterol, glucose, creatinine and other medical markers tested regularly over the past fifty-plus years.

The Dunedin Study is unique in that it has an incredible amount of data collected from a thousand people over a long period.

Professor Terrie Moffit and her team decided that they could use their own biomarkers which should be more accurate and valid than those used in other genetic clocks. They identified 173 DNA methylation marks and developed an algorithm which could accurately work out someone's biological age taken from the blood of a pin-prick blood test. This is called the Dunedin PACE algorithm with PACE standing for pace of ageing calculated from the epigenome.

So all of this DNA information is used to see what effect it has on the epigenome which controls everything your genes do. This gives a clear picture as to the amount of damage to your cells which has occurred at this particular time in a person's life.

What the blood test will tell us is how much damage has been done to your cells, which in turn tells us what your biological age is.

It also measures the length of our telomeres and, better still, it will actually tell you how fast you're ageing.

LOWERING YOUR OWN BIOLOGICAL AGE

All you have read so far deals with the biological and biochemical processes which take place within your body. The result of all of this activity will depend almost completely on how you live in and behave in your environment. If you live in a stressful environment, have a stressful job, eat all the wrong types of food and lead a sedentary lifestyle, your mind and body will suffer accordingly.

Although your DNA will not change, you will have out-of-control stress hormones, high blood sugar levels, are likely to be overweight and have a general lack of fitness. Your epigenomic system will have a difficult job sending out the right signals to your genes and your biochemistry generally will be out of whack.

Some of your genes will be switched on when they should be switched off and vice versa, and this will cause cellular damage over and above the normal wear and tear for your age. This can result in the early onset of serious health conditions like dementia, diabetes, Parkinson's disease, arthritis, heart disease and stroke.

Your rate of ageing will likely be too high, meaning that if this pattern continues you will become old before your time.

Thankfully, on the flipside of this, if you lead a relatively stress-free life, eat well and exercise regularly, your rate of ageing is likely to be quite low and you will remain young well into your old age.

Wouldn't that be nice? Well, the rest of this chapter is about finding simple ways to do exactly that. Before we do this, I would first like to revisit some of our super-agers and their polar opposites.

SUPER AGERS AND NOT SO SUPER

Earlier this year I had lunch with ninety-eight-year-old Margaret Borland. She greets me with a firm handshake, I can see the steely glint in her eye, and I know that she is still as fit as a fiddle.

She plays golf at Dunedin's Chisholm Park links twice a week, and of course she walks those nine holes. Jokingly, she says that she prays for rain every Tuesday and Thursday as her recent form hasn't been too flash.

Her garden is on a sloping section. That's no barrier to Margaret and she also walks regularly around her Anderson's Bay area.

Sharp as a tack mentally and playing bridge weekly, she recalls many names and details from her past life as a physio and national tennis champion.

We leave the cafe at our downtown Auckland location and encounter two steep flights of stairs on our way out. I look sideways at her enquiringly and soon have my answer as she walks quite briskly down them. Holding onto the handrail mind, she does admit to cutting herself a bit of slack these days.

As I have written about earlier, twenty-odd years earlier my wife Kate and I owned a thirty-four-bed rest home. My experience with most of our residents was at polar opposites to recent experiences with the phenomenal and inspiring group of oldies who are adding their stories to my book.

Some of our residents were in their late sixties and others only in their seventies. They had come to us as they were no longer able to cope in their own homes. They were dependent upon us to attend to nearly all of their needs. Meals, showering, drug administration, cleaning, bed-making and even toileting were all part of this.

Many were simply old before their time. These were very different from my fiercely independent recent group.

At both ends of this spectrum there are many clues and lessons to be learned. It is the difference between losing your independence earlier on, or gaining one, two or even three or more decades of bonus time living a fully independent and active lifestyle. In other words, extending your healthspan years exponentially.

Also very different would be the rate of ageing of both of these groups of people. The rest home group on average would have had a biological age higher than their real age. My recent group would be substantially lower.

Arch Jelley is 101 years old, still does 100 squats a day and walks about four kilometres on what is quite hilly country. Both he and Margaret look and act like people in their seventies.

On this basis, it would be quite feasible that their Dunedin PACE Value could be as low as 0.65. On the other hand, our residents could be on average 1.2 plus, putting them at risk of having a chronic disease. This was the case more often than not.

The PACE Value is the rate at which you age biologically. The lower the better, with a value of 1.0 being the actual rate of time itself; in a calendar year you would age biologically by twelve months.

At a PACE Value of 0.65 you would age 7.8 months biologically every calendar year. At a PACE Value of 1.2 you would age 14.4 months each calendar year.

About 80 per cent of your potential ageing and future health is about the choices you make in life, not your genes.

I rest my case; now let's take a look at how we can go about this.

TAKING THE FIRST STEP

If you have been thinking to yourself, well, maybe I should have a crack at this, a good first step would be to consider what I believe to be the ultimate motivation. It is quite simply to consider how incredible your own body is. I still remember vividly my afternoon at the Body Worlds exhibition. It was both awesome and inspiring to see all of these different cadavers minus their skins.

Google 'Body Worlds' (you may have done this before), and check out the incredible mix of bones, muscles, tendons, ligaments, nerves, blood vessels and much more. And, of course, your brain encased in that bony skull masterminding our every move.

Now relate all this back to your own body and remember that it is built just like one of Gunther von Hagen's models and is every bit as wonderful. Well, why would you not do your absolute best to look after what is your biggest asset? And this unique mix of trillions of cells is the only one you are ever going to get. This is a once-only opportunity!

There is nothing like being in good health and my mother often used to tell me this. Now I believe her.

When things are going well you don't even notice your body. It's just there. It's only when you have an accident or become unwell that your senses become immediately amplified and aware of the discomfort and pain.

Sometimes accidents are just unavoidable. Falling ill, as in getting Covid or a cold, is also usually beyond your control. There is one thing that is well within your control, however, and that is taking really good care of this incredible body you have been gifted with.

Remember that about 80 per cent of your future health will depend on your environment and how you behave in it. Only about 20 per cent is related to your inherited genes.

Your body takes care of you 24/7 day in, day out. Your heart never takes a break and pumps between 7000 and 8000 litres of blood around your body every day. In a year that's enough to fill an Olympic-sized swimming pool. How fantastic is that? Imagine that. You've also got your own food-processing plant and waste disposal unit, also operating 24/7.

As I am writing this, my brain is performing myriad tasks to allow me to come up with these sentences, let alone all the other complex operations keeping me upright in my chair and allowing my fingers to tap away on this keyboard.

Biochemical miracles are routinely performed to keep you alive and well. Mitochondria are like bustling factories providing energy for your cells. Your stem cells beaver away renewing your cells as others die. Nutrient sensors cleverly distribute food and drink to the best possible places. Protein provides you with amino acids which are helping to build muscles, tendons, ligaments and all the other structures in your body.

All of this incredible non-stop activity is highly dependent on you behaving in a way which is in keeping with what your human body is set up for. Eating well, hydrating regularly, keeping your body moving and living a relatively stress-free life are some of the basics we have been talking about.

If you are subjecting your body regularly to unhealthy foods, a lack of exercise and high stress levels, your clever body will only be able to compensate for some of this negative stuff for a while.

There is a limit to this, and once you cross this line, cell damage will occur and your biological age will increase sometimes way more than it should.

REVERSING DAMAGE

It's your choice. The good news is that cell damage can be reversed by changes to your environment and the way you behave in it.

Remember that on average people only reach their mid-sixties before they get a chronic illness. By making the right lifestyle choices you could stay healthy for an extra decade or more.

Think back a decade to what you were doing and some of the things that you have done. It's a great deal of healthy living that you can fit into a decade.

The goal is to keep your cells as young as possible.

Are you ready?

Part Three
THE DON'T ACT YOUR AGE CHALLENGE
A Life-changing Challenge!

The Don't Act Your Age Challenge is all about forming new lifestyle habits to increase your years of healthy life

HOW IT WORKS

1. Raise awareness – This can be quite wide-ranging and includes discovering problem areas in your life and the ways in which new lifestyle habits could help.
2. Gain clarity – Providing simple and practical guidelines to help understand 'the nature of the beast'.
3. Make changes.
4. Practise these changes daily where possible and review your progress regularly. To do this just simply ask yourself open-ended questions like 'How am I going?' or

'What can I do here?' This encourages you to check your progress and find answers if you need to.
5. Establish new lifestyle habits. Two months of conscious practice is about what is needed to make the changes become a habit.
6. Beware of basic human nature which can cause you to slip up and revert to where you were. Continue to be aware of and review your new habits. After a while you'll have them for life. Just like you brush your teeth!

If you trust the process, believe that it is totally doable and if you are ready to make a few permanent changes, you'll succeed. Your future health will benefit from these new habits and sometimes these will prove to be life changing.

HOW TO GO ABOUT YOUR CHALLENGE

Your first step is to put aside the time to read through the challenge. This will help you to become aware of any area where you think you need to make changes.

Take little steps and make your selected changes into permanent habits. When you have succeeded with this method for one habit, this will give you the confidence to add new habits as you see fit.

Because your **physical functionality** is so important I suggest that you give this top priority and do the physical tests first to see what you need to work on. Make notes on what stretches and exercises you are going to include in your routine.

Nutrition is also a top priority, so start small by picking two or three things you want to change. This could be to change your cereal and bread and cut down on sushi rolls. Just these three will make a big difference to your daily tally of teaspoons of sugar.

Hydration, breaking up long sitting periods and building resilience are the other three. Don't try for too many changes at once; if you see room for improvement, just focus on one change at a time and make each one stick.

Atomic habits – A unique and effective way to build all of your different habit changes into your often busy days is to simply attach tiny habits to your daily existing habits. The concept has been developed by American author and presenter James Clear, and he has written a best-seller by the same name.

The following are a few examples:

Balance
Stand on one leg while brushing your teeth.
When walking, walk along any painted lines or kerbs.
Agility
Put on a catchy tune while waiting for your dinner to cook and do a little dance around.
Fitness
Always take the stairs.
When walking, add in some hilly bits.
Flexibility
Do some stretches while watching TV.
Do head and neck stretches while microwaving your rolled oats.
Strength
Do press-ups or planks while watching TV.
Do squats while out walking.

Once you have selected what your various new daily habits are, we will take you through a process to attach them to some of your existing habits.

Welcome to the challenge. I hope that you will enjoy the process, develop some new lifestyle habits and gain some extra years of good health.

The challenge has five separate habits to focus on:

1. Improving physical functionality
2. Nutrition
3. Hydration
4. Breaking up long periods of inactive sitting
5. Building resilience

1
IMPROVING PHYSICAL FUNCTIONALITY (PF)

This is broken up into three parts. The first is to clarify what this is all about, the second to put you through a series of physical tests, and the third to work out a programme for you to improve any areas of weakness you might have.

Remember the BAFFS acronym covers all aspects of your physical abilities. They are balance, agility, fitness (cardiovascular), flexibility and strength. Collectively these are at the heart of your PF, especially as you grow older.

Your very independence relies on you having sufficient balance to avoid falls, agility to sidestep imminent disasters, enough cardiovascular puff to climb up stairs, good flexibility and sufficient strength to cope with your day-to-day physical needs.

UNDERSTANDING AND TESTING YOUR BAFFS

This whole area of BAFFS is very wide. To give you some clarity we will start by giving you a simple big-picture look at how it all fits together.

Your arms, hands, legs and feet tend to naturally take a fair bit of your daily exercise load. Whether you are walking, doing housework, cooking, gardening, playing cards or any other leisure activity, your limbs and their appendages are kept pretty busy. This is why I want to first focus on the rest of your body, of which key parts are often sadly neglected.

Your core runs from and includes the pelvic floor up to where the ribs begin. I have invented a new term which we will call the **upper core** which runs from the bottom of the ribs to the top of the neck.

Most people's height reduces by up to seven and a half centimetres (three inches) over their lifetimes. That is the height of an average teacup. Or really high heels!

Most of this height loss occurs over the length of the spine. The discs between the vertebrae flatten and the spaces between bones become smaller. And gravity also plays its part with its constant downward pull.

Osteoporosis, which is where the bones become less dense, will also contribute to a loss of height.

Much of this height loss can be avoided by strengthening the muscles, tendons, ligaments and cartilage of the core and upper core.

And in turn, these exercises will also help strengthen bones and prevent osteoporosis.

Your core and upper core are powerhouses which provide stability and strength for all parts of our body. We will cover specific exercises for these later in this chapter.

The BAFFS are:

Balance – Unless you are sitting down, any physical activity requires balance in varying degrees. As we have discussed earlier, your ability to stay balanced in a variety of different activities will largely depend on how strong your muscles and skeletal system are.

Agility – Physically, it is your ability to move your feet and your body quickly and easily. Mentally it is your ability to think and react quickly to any given situation which requires you to move. Your agility is tested in any activity which requires rapid movement like skipping, hopping, racquet sports, contact sports, hopscotch and many more.

Fitness (cardiovascular) – This is any activity which helps you to get puffing and your heart and lungs pumping.

Flexibility – The ability of your body to easily adapt without pain or stress to any particular position that is required in your day-to-day living. As you age, yoga and other passive stretching exercises will help your body to retain its flexibility.

Strength – Your strength is the physical energy that you have, which gives you the ability to perform various actions, such as lifting or moving things. Your goal would be to retain your strength throughout your life. And even beyond the expectations of your actual age.

MEASURING YOUR OWN BAFFS CAPABILITIES

We have put together different physical tests, many taken from normal daily activities, to test your own capabilities. This should give you a good indication of where you stand and what you need to do.

Safety is the key – Your first consideration is to stay safe. If you are not confident of carrying out any one of these tests and think may injure yourself, give it a miss.

We will separate our test into five categories, one for each of the BAFFS. Some of these activities will engage two or more BAFFS. For example, star jumps are a good all-rounder requiring balance, agility, cardio fitness and strength.

Balance

1. Stand on one leg for ten seconds without putting your other foot on the ground. One point
2. Stand on one leg and close your eyes for five seconds without putting your other foot on the ground. Two points
3. Stand on tiptoes for five seconds. One point
4. Stand on tiptoes for ten seconds with your eyes closed. Two points
5. Stand with feet together, place the heel of your right foot directly in front of the toes of your left foot. Repeat by placing the heel of your left foot in front of the toes of your right foot. Repeat this heel to toe placement six times without stopping. Put your arms out to the side to help with balance. One point
6. Walk on a raised kerb for ten metres. You must stay on the kerb. Two points
7. Put a pair of shorts on while standing. One point
8. Put a sock on one foot while standing. Two points

Agility

1. Stand on one leg and hop on the spot five times. One point

2. Stand on one leg and hop five times on each leg. Ten hops in total. Two points
3. Stand with feet together beside a line. Keeping feet together, jump from one side of the line to the other five times. One point
4. Stand with feet together beside a line. Keeping feet together, jump from one side of the line to the other ten times. Two points
5. Hold a tennis ball in one hand and throw it above head height and catch it with the other hand. Repeat five times without missing. One point
6. Hold a tennis ball in one hand and throw it up and over your head and catch with two hands behind your back. You need to have one successful catch out of three attempts. Two points
7. Skipping with a rope. Skip continuously for ten seconds. One point
8. Skip continuously for twenty seconds. Two points

Note: If a rope is not available, do your skips without a rope. Each skip is two hops on one leg followed by two hops on the opposite leg, all in one continuous movement.

Ten skips moving forward is one point. Ten skips moving forward followed by ten skips moving backward to your starting point is two points.

Fitness – cardiovascular

These exercises should be carried out one after the other with a minute's break between each one.

1. Star jumps. Standing, hands by your sides, jump feet apart while bringing arms straight above your head into a handclap. Jump back to the starting position and repeat five times. One point
2. Star jumps as above, repeat fifteen times. Two points
3. Squat-thrusts (burpees). Standing feet together, put hands on floor in front of you, and jump your feet back into press-up position, jump feet back to between your hands and stand up. This should be a continuous movement. Repeat three times. One point
4. Squat-thrusts as above, repeat ten times. Two points
5. Step-ups. Find a nearby step, and step up with one foot, bring the other foot up to the step and down with one after the other foot. Repeat this five times. One point
6. Step-ups as above, repeat fifteen times at pace. Two points
7. Stairs. Climb up and down three flights of stairs, using the handrail if necessary. One point
8. Stairs. Climb up and down five flights of stairs. Two points

Flexibility

1. Cutting or trimming your own toenails. If, at the time of doing this test series you are able to cut your own toenails, this will count as two points.
2. Back touch test. Put your right hand over your shoulder to touch your back. Bring your left hand up your back to touch the fingers of your right hand. One point

3. Reverse this same test using your left hand over your shoulder and your right hand up your back to touch the other hand. One point
4. Touching your toes. From a standing position with straight legs, touch your toes with your fingers. Two points
5. Seated reach test. From a sitting position with your legs out straight and wide apart, touch your toes with fingers of both hands. One point
6. From the same position with your feet together, touch your toes. Two points
7. Neck stretch. You need help with this one. From standing, without turning your shoulders get a partner to measure the distance your chin moves when you turn it as far as you can to the right from a central position. You can also repeat the test to the left to see if they are similar. Ten centimetres is one point. Thirteen centimetres plus is two points.

Strength

Press-ups

For a press-up you must have a straight back. Each press-up goes from having straight arms down to your nose almost touching the floor and back to straight arms.

1. Men – one point for ten press-ups, two points for fifteen press-ups
2. Women – one point for fifteen press-ups with your knees on the ground, two points for ten regular press-ups

Dips

With the heels of your hands on the edge of a chair and feet out the front, dip your backside towards the floor until the angle of your upper and lower arms are at about ninety degrees. Pull up to your starting position. Ten dips, one point. Twenty dips, two points.

Note: If you cannot manage dips off the back of a chair, you can do ten using your kitchen bench (which is higher) for one point.

Planking

On your front, with body straight and supported on your elbows and lower arms and toes. Holding for fifteen seconds – one point. The same exercise holding for thirty seconds – two points.

If you cannot manage a full plank, support yourself on your knees, holding for sixty seconds – one point.

Chair stands

Use a standard chair with a back. Sit with your back touching the back of the chair. Have your arms folded against your chest. One chair stand is to fully stand and return to the same position. See how many you can do in thirty seconds.

1. Men – one point for sixteen, two points for nineteen
2. Women – one point for fourteen, two points for seventeen

You will now have an idea of what your strengths and weaknesses are. The next section will give you all you need to concentrate on your weaknesses and improve your overall physical functionality.

WORKING OUT A BAFFS IMPROVEMENT PLAN FOR YOU

The idea here is to come up with a short routine of a few minutes that you can do each day. And you will be able to do this in your lounge at home, or hotel or motel room while you are away.

You can break up this routine into smaller bits using the 'Atomic Habits' principle and attach these to some of your regular daily habits.

This routine should have emphasis on your weaknesses and at the same time include elements of all of the five BAFFS. This routine will supplement all of the other physical activities that you take part in and ensure that all bases are covered.

You can use my notes on each of the BAFFS in the following pages and any of the tests that you did earlier to put your routine together. You will find an example of how to put this together using Atomic Habits at the end of this chapter.

Once you have been doing this routine daily for a couple of months it will have become a habit and part of your daily routine. Just like brushing your teeth.

Balance

Retaining your ability to easily go up and down stairs and steps, and generally prevent yourself from falling, is a crucial part of being able to maintain your independence.

Stand on one leg: The simplest and safest way to improve balance is to practise standing on one leg in a number of different ways.

You can put your other leg out to either side or to the front or back. This has the added benefit of helping to improve other muscle groups. For example, standing on one leg with your other leg out to the side helps to strengthen the adductor muscles in the groin.

Walk heel to toe: The other excellent exercise is to walk heel to toe for a few metres. Hold your arms out to the side to help with balance. Start by putting your heel in front of your other foot so it just touches your big toe and keep repeating this.

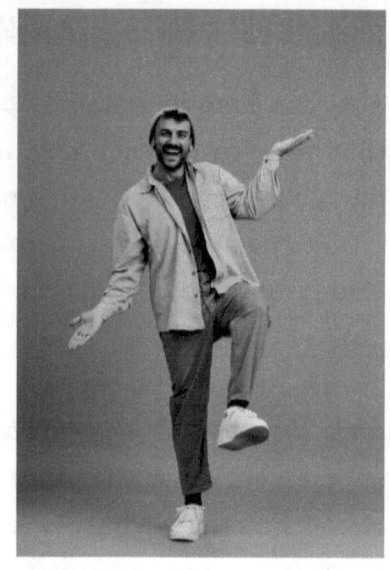

These balance exercises help your brain to form new connections and strengthen the coordination between different parts of your body. In recognising these new activities, your joints and muscles will send messages to the brain which will help to rewire it and to improve your balance.

Agility

Agility is really your ability to move your body easily and quickly into a variety of positions. Being more agile will help you to retain your balance should anything potentially dangerous unexpectedly come your way. For example, it could be your dog on a lead pulling you off balance, or avoiding that pesky kid on a skateboard.

Dance, skip, hop: The earlier tests will give you a variety of options for agility exercises. Another way to get your feet and body moving naturally is to dance to your favourite piece of music. Whatever it is, skipping, hopping or dancing, it will all help you to become more agile.

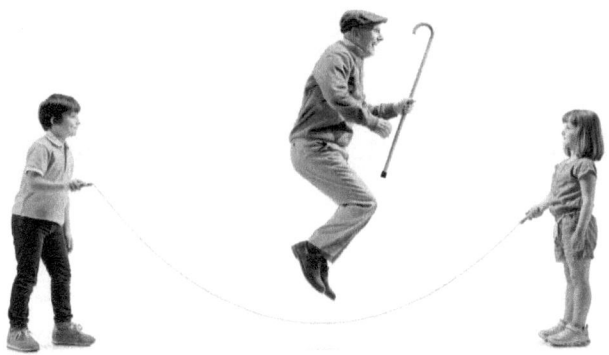

Getting up off the ground: This is a key skill in being able to retain your independence and well worth practising daily. It is not only your agility that is being tested. Elements of flexibility and strength are also required.

Sit on the floor with your knees bent, rotate your body so that one knee is on the ground. Try this on both sides to discover which side is the most comfortable. Turn so that you can put your other foot beside the knee on the ground.

Keep turning and place your hands shoulder width apart on the ground in front of your hip on this same side.

Keep rotating the same way and this same hip should be able to come off the ground sufficiently for you to be able to be up on your hand and knees.

From this position you should be able to make your way to your feet.

There are free YouTube videos which you can access to get a better picture of different techniques for safely getting down and up from the ground.

If you struggle to get up off the ground, you should practise this technique regularly.

Side shuffles: These two are excellent low-impact and safe exercises if you are just starting out to improve your agility from scratch.

The first one is stand feet together, step to the right, feet together, step to the right, feet together and reverse back to the starting position.

In the second one, do exactly the same except with each step you put your stepping foot in front of the other one so you are crossing over each time.

Repeat these a few times and perhaps speed up the pace as you improve.

Fitness (cardiovascular)

Once again, use the guidelines in the tests with the general idea being to do short bursts of high-intensity exercise at your own level of fitness.

This may be a combination of, say, twenty-five star jumps, followed by ten squat-thrusts and fifty air punches while jogging on the spot. Take a minute's break between each set.

Climbing up and down flights of stairs is an excellent way to get you puffing and with the additional benefit of giving your legs and gluteals a good workout.

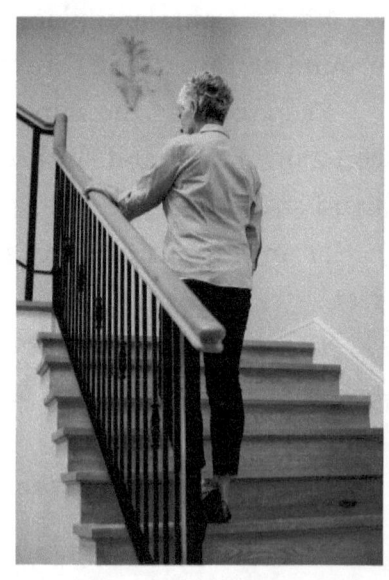

You can do these as part of your daily routine and also after you have had a prolonged time sitting down. If I have been playing bridge for a couple of hours, I will always do a short cardio routine and perhaps some strength exercises as well.

These short daily bursts are a great addition to any other physical activities that you are involved in.

Flexibility

One area which often misses out is that of flexibility, which is primarily gained by passive stretching. This is where particular stretches are held in one position for a short period of time. Yoga and Pilates are good examples of this.

Regular stretching is a non-negotiable discipline. You absolutely do not want to lose flexibility in key areas like the neck, shoulders and hips. Once this happens, your tendons, ligaments and cartilage become brittle and weakened, and your ability to perform simple daily tasks can be severely compromised.

Just as you brush your teeth, ideally stretching should become a daily activity.

The following are basic stretches which I use and will cover most of the key muscle groups and joints of the body.

Neck, triceps, shoulder and upper back stretch: This is in four movements. With one arm straight and above your head, drop your hand back till it touches your shoulder. Take your other hand and hold your elbow. With this hand pull your elbow directly backwards and hold for a few seconds. Repeat this movement with the other arm. Hold each one for about ten seconds.

Roll both your shoulders back and around in a circular movement four times.

Turn your chin as far round towards your right shoulder as you can and repeat with the movement towards the left shoulder. Hold for about ten seconds in each direction.

Gently rotate your head around your neck in a circular movement one way then the other

Repeat the sequence of these four movements at least three

times.

Benefits – Most of us will at some time or other experience stiffness and soreness around the head, neck, shoulders and upper back. That feeling of 'oh my God my head feels too heavy for my neck to support it'. One set of muscles run from the cervical spine and insert into the lower part of our skull. If they become tight, this can result in headaches and a sore and stiff neck. This is only one of a number of sets of muscle groups in this key upper part of your body.

This set of four stretches will help to stretch and keep supple all of the muscles and other soft tissues in your head, neck, shoulders and upper back. I have used this brilliant foursome daily now for many years and they have really helped to relieve stiffness and tension.

Spine, lower back, hips, hamstrings and calf stretch: This is another good all-rounder.

Feet wide apart and legs straight, arms folded. Drop your folded arms slowly down towards the floor and hold for three to four breaths.

Repeat three to five times.

Benefits – This is a powerful stretch for all of the muscle groups and areas mentioned above.

Child's Pose: Kneel on the floor with your knees apart and sit back on your heels. Lean forward so your stomach touches your thighs, and rest your forehead on the floor. You can extend your arms out in front of you with your palms down, or place them by your sides or under your forehead.

Benefits – This is a good all-rounder for stretching shoulders, lower back and hips.

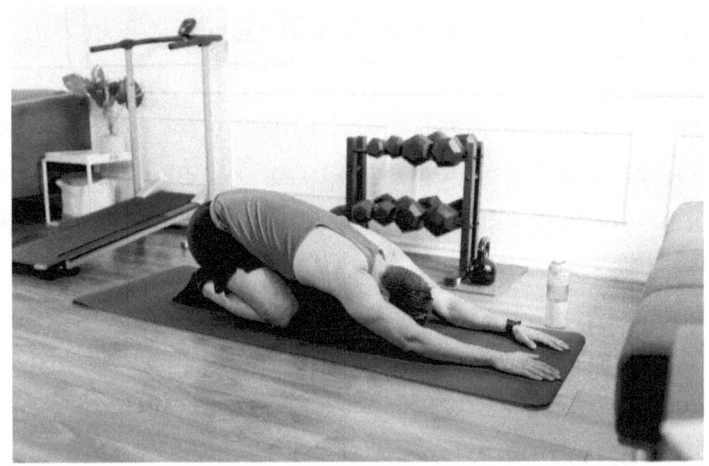

Lower back and hips: Lie on your back with your legs straight, grasp your right knee in both hands and pull up as far as you can towards your chest and hold for ten to fifteen seconds. Repeat using the other leg.

Lie on your back and resting on your elbows. Leaving your backside on the floor, gently push your hips towards your feet. You will feel your lumbar spine (which is the area just above your pelvis) arch slightly.

Gently push your hips back to your starting position and try to push your lumbar spine into the floor.

Gently repeat these movements a number of times. Try to get the feeling of arching the lumbar spine and then reversing this.

You can do this same exercise by standing with your back to the wall and your heels about three to five centimetres from the wall.

You can arch the spine and then push it back into the wall by simply leaving your bum where it is against the wall and bending your knees to get the arch and up on your toes to push your spine back into the wall.

I prefer the standing option. Try both and select the one that works for you.

Benefits – The lumbar spine and hips are part of your core, and lower back pain is a common problem. When I finished physical education teaching at age forty-one, I often had lower back pain and was as stiff as a board in this area. These sets of exercises helped me to re-educate this area and gradually gain back my flexibility. If you are anything like me, you will need to be patient. My progress was slow and I had to keep at it for quite a while. They are now part of my daily stretching routine.

Downward Dog: This is simply one of the best stretches for multiple parts of the body including shoulders, spine, hips, hamstrings and calves. A staple of most yoga programmes.

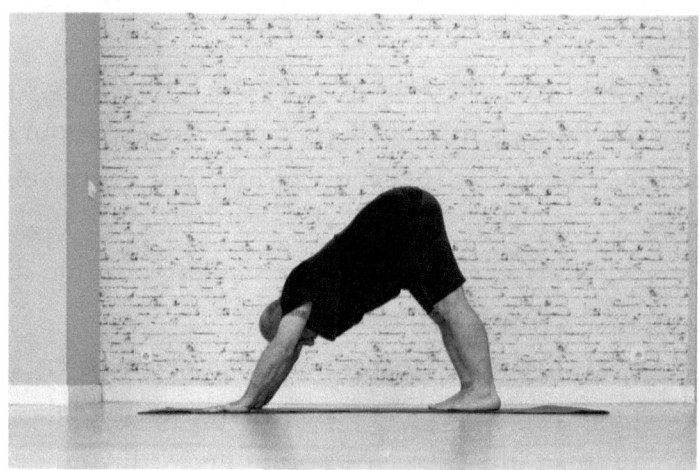

On hands and knees, raise your buttocks and at the same time straighten your legs while keeping your heels flat on the ground. Push your buttocks up as high as possible and hold for fifteen to twenty seconds. Your head should stay in line between your arms.

At first you may not be able to keep your heels flat on the ground.

In time, as you become more flexible, you may be able to achieve this.

Benefits – As I have mentioned, this famous yoga pose stretches multiple areas of the body and would be one of the first stretches included in any routine.

Calf and Achilles tendon stretch: You can perform this by placing both hands against a wall or bench at about kitchen bench height. With straight legs and feet together, walk your feet back until your heels are off the ground.

Push your heels back to touch the ground and hold for ten to fifteen seconds. Increase the intensity of the stretch by pushing your hips towards the ground.

You can also do this with one leg back at a time. Repeat five to ten times.

Benefits – Your calves and the Achilles strap-like tendon wrapping around your heel are key in most movements of the foot and leg. This simple stretch will help ensure that they remain flexible and not prone to injury. If you have experienced or ever seen anyone receive an Achilles separation, you will know the sheer incapacity it causes.

Windscreen Wipers: Lie on your back with your arms fully extended out to the side with the backs of your hands on the floor. Bring both knees up together towards your chest. With the backs of your hands still on the floor, rotate your knees to one side or the other as far as you can towards the ground then repeat on the other side. Repeat ten times.

You may find it easier to do this same exercise keeping your feet on the ground.

Benefits – This is a great all-round core exercise engaging abdominals, hip flexors and gluteals.

Summary: Once you have become familiar with these stretches you will find that they take about five to ten minutes to complete. I try to do two of these sets every day. If at any time I feel stiffness in any of these areas, I will do the appropriate stretch.

Retaining your skeletal flexibility will allow you to ward off much of the normal stiffness and pain that you experience in your later years. This is a crucial part of the challenge to get the best out of the rest of your life.

Strength

As I mentioned, your arms and legs tend to get a reasonable workout with the normal daily demands of your life. Sometimes the core and upper core (your trunk) miss out. Regular specific strength exercises can prevent deterioration of this all-important core of your body.

If you can retain a strong core as you age, this will help to prevent osteoporosis, muscle weakening and deterioration of other soft tissues.

You will notice that many people as they grow older become more stooped, with shoulders slumping forward and their head and neck tending to also bend forward. This is often the result of a loss of core strength. It is really difficult to hold your head up nice and straight if your upper spine and neck muscles are weak.

This is the same problem if your shoulders are slumping forward and not held back in a more upright position. This position means that your spine is also bent forward.

Right down through your lower core areas to your pelvic floor, the same rules apply.

These following specific strength exercises, if performed regularly, will ensure that you can defy your chronological age by having an erect posture and strong core even into your advanced years. Two of these are a repeat of exercises you saw in our BAFFS series of tests.

Crunches: lie on your back with your knees bent and anchored under a couch, bed or bench. Cross your arms across your chest and gently roll your shoulders up off the ground and down again.

For a start I would just do a few of these, otherwise you might end up with rather sore abdominals.

Gradually build up to whatever you are comfortable with. Three sets of ten with a rest in between would be sufficient.

Benefits – Crunches are a classic core exercise. They specifically target your abdominal muscles. They will also strengthen the oblique muscles on either side of your abdominals and muscles in your pelvis and lower back.

At the time of writing this, I had completely forgotten about the all-round brilliance of these powerhouse crunches. Having jogged my memory, I will be adding a few of these to my own routine.

Press-ups: For press-ups you must have a straight back. Each press-up goes from having straight arms down to your nose almost touching the floor and back to straight arms.

If you cannot manage a press-up, do them with your knees on the ground. They will still benefit the same muscle groups. You may be able to work your way up to the full press-up version.

Benefits – They strengthen the lower back and other parts of the core, triceps, pectorals and shoulders. Press-ups are another great all-round strength exercise. Once again, start off by doing a few and concentrating on having good

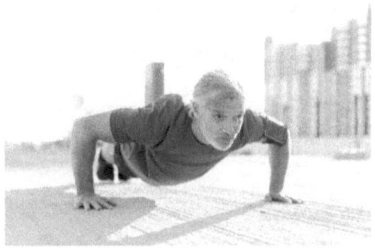

form. You are better to do just a few press-ups with good form as detailed above than a lot of half-hearted ones.

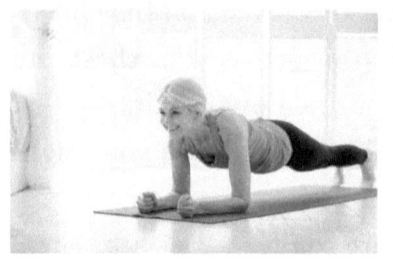

Planking: Lie on your front, with body straight and supported on your elbows and lower arms and toes.

You can have your fingers lightly interlaced and your hands and elbows forming a triangle shape.

If you cannot manage a full plank, support yourself on your knees.

For a start, only hold the position for as long as you are comfortable. Ten to thirty seconds would be about right. You can progress from there if you feel the need.

Benefits – Planking helps to stabilise the lumbar spine and pelvis. And it strengthens the abdominal and gluteal (buttocks) muscles.

Bridges: A bridge is a simple exercise with a number of benefits.

Lie on your back with your knees bent. Raise your buttocks off the ground for a few seconds.

Repeat at least five times.

Benefits – Bridging engages core muscles, particularly gluteals, and also your quadriceps (thigh) muscles.

Opposite arm and leg raise: From on all fours, raise your right hand and left leg off the ground at the same time. Do this movement slowly and extend both your arm and leg as much as possible if your balance allows this.

Repeat using opposite hand and leg. Hold each movement for a few seconds and repeat ten times.

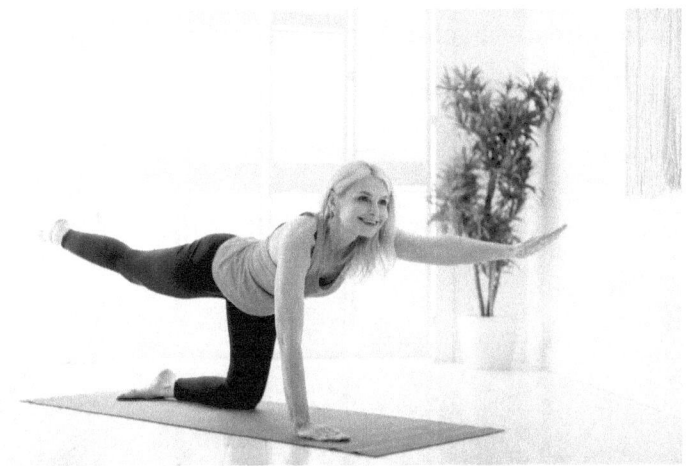

Benefits – This is a great all-round core exercise and helps to strengthen your abdomen, lower back, hip flexors, and spine. And it has an excellent balance factor.

Summary – Having a strong core and upper core will ensure that you will have good posture and be able to easily cope with your day-to-day physical challenges well into later life. This is a must to help both lower your biological age and increase your healthspan years.

Arms and legs

As we have mentioned earlier, your limbs get a reasonable workout just going about your normal daily routine. A few muscle groups need to be mentioned as they sometimes get neglected or can benefit from some specific resistance exercises.

Arms

Triceps – Located at the back of your upper arm. Your biceps get most of the action in lifting anything, and triceps by comparison are left relatively unemployed. Over the years they tend to become smaller and weaker, and this becomes quite obvious with the floppy wings that can appear in our upper arms.

Dips have already been mentioned and will help to strengthen this important muscle group.

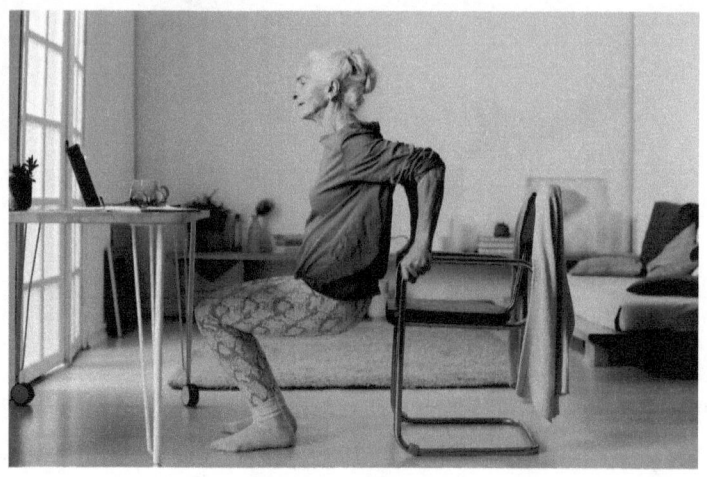

If you are not strong enough to do dips, you can use a stretchy band or a dumbbell. The action is to hold the dumbbell above your head and lower down towards the back of your shoulder and up again.

With a stretchy band, hold one end in each hand above your head and the band under your shoulders. Lower both hands down towards the back of your shoulder and up again.

You can also use the dumbbells or the stretchy bands for biceps or wrist curls.

Grip strength – As you grow older your continuing ability to perform basic functional tasks around your house and garden becomes important, e.g. opening cans and bottles. You can improve your grip strength by regularly squeezing balls. Soft balls smaller than a tennis ball and bigger than a squash ball are ideal.

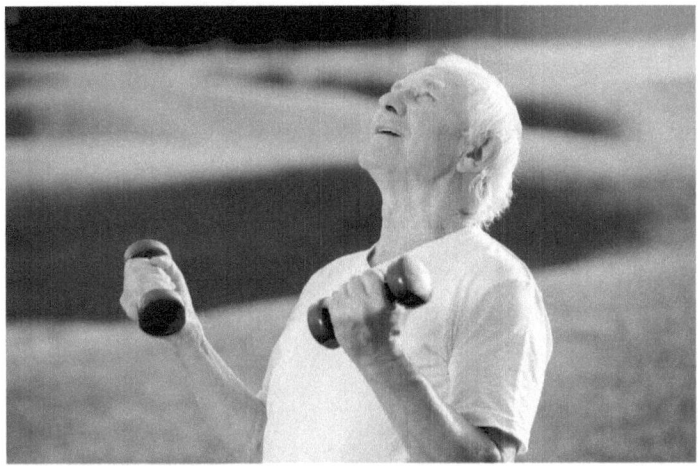

Legs

If you feel that your leg muscles need strengthening, squats are excellent for this. They work on your large thigh muscles (quadriceps). Use calf-raises for strengthening your lower leg.

If you are walking regularly and active in other ways, your legs are getting daily workouts which should keep muscle, joint and soft tissues in good shape as you grow older.

SUMMARY

You can include any of the above stretches and exercises in the flexibility and strength areas that we have just covered in your regular routine. You can also go back to the physical tests in the previous chapter and include any of them in your regular routine.

Ideally, from all these different tests, stretches and other exercises you will be able to put together a daily routine of about ten to fifteen minutes. This routine should have a particular emphasis on areas of your BAFFS that you are weak in.

To reduce the need to do a ten to fifteen-minute separate routine, use the Atomic Habits concept to attach any of these exercises and stretches to your existing daily habits. This means that you can perform all of your different exercises and stretches throughout your day by attaching them to your existing daily habits.

You will probably already have physical activities that you take part in and will now have a good idea where they fit into the BAFFS scheme of things. Many activities and sports like walking, jogging, skiing, racquet sports, swimming and contact sports cover most of the BAFFS.

The idea of having a daily routine is to complement any of these other regular activities you take part in to ensure that you have all of the BAFFS covered. And to ensure that you are attending to your BAFFS on days where you are reasonably inactive.

2
NUTRITION

Although 'you are what you eat' may be a hackneyed old saying, it is very true. *If you eat and drink well, you are much more likely to have a healthy life than if you eat and drink badly.* In the latter case, you will almost certainly suffer ill health far earlier in life than you need to.

After selling our rest home in 2002, I acquired a life-coaching qualification and started my own life and business coaching practice. Many of my clients' goals were based around weight loss and before long the majority of my work was in this area.

This morphed into a business called Eat For Keeps (EFK) which helped people with weight and diabetes issues.

Over the next twenty years the EFK programme was used extensively by staff of major companies like dairy products giant Fonterra and New World Supermarkets. We received many referrals from medical practices, and a number of successful wellness challenges were carried out with at-risk patients.

I have had two books published on this subject and sold out the first print runs. Many testimonials have been received from business leaders, doctors, other health professionals and clients. And EFK's successes generated strong media interest over a long period.

Despite this, like any small business in a crowded market, we couldn't convert this success into a scalable business. I have found this incredibly frustrating. There is such a massive need for a solution in this critical area. If we could have scaled up our few thousand success stories exponentially, our method could have had a significant impact.

To know how to make the right food choices anytime, anywhere, you first need to gain some clarity as to what nutrition is all about. This is exactly what our approach does. It also provides the tools for people to gain the necessary skills and know-how to navigate the challenges of any food-service outlet they might visit.

With clarity comes confidence and the ability to take ownership and responsibility. This new, enlightened DIY spirit leads to great outcomes. Some of these have been life changing.

I am delighted to be able to include in this challenge a very simple and practical programme that we call 'The EFK Method'.

This can be read and digested in about an hour. Make notes on any changes that you would like to make to your eating habits and nutrition.

WELCOME TO 'THE EFK METHOD'

EFK's simple 'big picture' of nutrition

- All food and drink = 3 main nutrients, protein, fat and carbohydrate (PFCs), plus water and small amounts of vitamins and minerals.
- 'PFCs' do the big stuff like – Protein builds muscles, ligaments and other body tissues, fat regulates body temperature, and carbohydrate provides glucose for energy.
- Processed foods will contain different combinations of the above and also contain preservatives, flavourings and other additives mainly to help preserve shelf life. These additives provide no food value.
- All food and drink will have different combinations of PFCs.

A physiological process you need to know.

- During digestion carbohydrate makes the sugar glucose, for energy. If you exceed the amount you need the excess is stored as fat.
- A clever hormone called insulin, carries the glucose to where it is needed by the body. Over the years if we continue to exceed the amount of glucose we need, two things happen.
- One, your body becomes resistant to the insulin and you need more of it to shift the same amount of glucose.

- Two, your pancreas which makes the insulin cannot keep up with the demand.
- When this happens, the glucose remains in your blood-vessels, and damages them, causing life-threatening outcomes like stroke, heart disease, diabetes and amputations.

The PFC Table

It's vital that you understand what the protein, fat, carbohydrate content is of the food you usually eat. Although these tables will give you a useful guide, they are not complete.

- **Simple/Starchy carbohydrates** – Sugar, sweets, white bread products, baked goods (cakes, slices, biscuits, scones and muffins), processed breakfast cereals, sweet potato (kumara), potato, parsnips, most rice varieties, fruit juice and fizzy drinks.
- **Complex Carbohydrates** – Whole wheat and grainy breads, pasta, wholegrain almond and buckwheat flours, rolled oats, basmati and wild rice, green vegetables, citrus and temperate fruits, e.g. apples and peaches, legumes including chickpeas and lentils.
- **Protein-rich foods** – Beans and legumes.
- **Protein and fat-rich foods** – Meat, fish, seafood, eggs, nuts, seeds and dairy products.
- **Fat-rich foods** – Avocados and oils

Top Tips

- Simple and starchy food is either made from fast-digesting ingredients, like sugar and flour, or they are starchy foods like potatoes, kumara and rice. They make lots of glucose quickly, and include baked goods like muffins, scones and cakes, and all white bread products. You need to consume these in small quantities.
- Complex carbohydrate foods include green vegetables and fruit. They are firm textured, have lots of fibre, and will keep you fuller for longer by making glucose over a much longer period.
- Remember, that protein and fat-rich foods like fish and meat do not contain carbohydrate and have no effect on your blood-sugar levels.

The Glucose Equation

Now that you know that too much glucose is the problem, and that it comes from carbohydrate, you are probably wondering how much glucose you need.

- Harvard University have invented the perfect tool called the Glycaemic Load (GL) and for simplicities sake it can be measured in a form that you will be very familiar with, teaspoons of sugar (tsp).
- Each day we need to consume a maximum of between 20 – 30 tsp. These come from both added sugar and sugar that comes from the food after it has been digested.
- The number of tsp can vary according to your circumstances. A type 2 diabetic would need to consume

fewer tsp whereas a professional rugby player would need a much higher number.

The following meal and snack examples will give you a much clearer picture of what you need to do. Each time the first example is too high and the second is about right with an explanation to follow.

Note: These are estimates only. We don't count the protein and fat-rich foods like fish, meat and dairy products as they contain no carbohydrate and make zero tsp. Or count very small quantities like the small amount of jam on a piece of toast. All totals rounded off to the nearest number.

Breakfast 1 – Cornflakes, milk, yoghurt, half a banana, one piece of white toast, with jam, coffee, with one sugar = 14 tsp
Breakfast 2 – Porridge, teaspoon of honey, milk, one piece of heavy grain bread with avocado, cup of tea = 3 tsp
Cornflakes versus rolled oats. The former is light and crunchy and contains up to 75% simple carbs. Rolled oats is about 50% complex carbs and has slow-digesting grains. 8.8 v 0.9 tsp.
White toast at 3.2 v 1.8 tsp for the grain bread. Half a banana = 1.8 tsp.
Morning tea 1 – A small muffin and a cup of tea with one sugar = 9 tsp.
Morning tea 2 – Mandarin with a few almond nuts = 3 tsp.
The muffin makes 8.2 tsp and the sugar 1 tsp. The mandarin 3 and the nuts 0 tsp. The muffin has high levels of white-flour full of fast-digesting simple carbs.
Lunch 1 – 4 x sushi rolls and a glass of orange juice = 14 tsp
Lunch 2 – 2 x poached eggs on heavy, grain bread toast, a flat white = 2 tsp

Each Sushi roll produces 2.6 tsp because of its sticky white rice. The fruit juice 3.5 tsp. Whereas poached eggs and avo are 0, and grain bread 1.8 tsp.

Afternoon tea 1 – an apple = 1 tsp.

Afternoon tea 2 – Oat cake biscuit, with pickle and cheese = 1 tsp. Both good choices although the second option is more balanced in that it contains protein fat and carbs.

Dinner 1 – A steak with a large helping of mashed potato and green vegetables, with a small white bread roll = 13 tsp

Dinner 2 – Pan fried salmon, with a small potato and green vegetables with aioli sauce = 4 tsp

Both the steak and salmon and green vegetables make zero tsp. The small potato makes 4 tsp while the large portion of starchy, mashed spuds make 7 and the bread roll 6.5 tsp.

Summing Up

- Option 1's total tsp of sugar for the day were 51 which is far too high, while the second option total was 13. The first option had a high level of simple and starchy carbs, the second was focussed more on protein and fat-rich foods and could probably have had a bit of an increase in carbs.
- Remember that foods like meat, fish, seafood, dairy products, nuts and seeds and avo are protein and fat-rich and contain no carbs, therefore make zero tsp of sugar.
- Just keep the simple and starchy carbohydrate food and drinks like rice, cakes, slices, muffins, scones, biscuits, potato, kumara, fruit juice and fizzy drinks down to a minimum. And, always eat them together with more

sustaining food. Keep your phone handy if you need to check your tables.

Table of tsp of Sugar Values

Bread (65g or two slices of sandwich thickness)

- Wholegrain 3.5
- Sourdough 3.8
- Wholemeal 5.6
- White bread products, e.g. bagels, buns, focaccia 6.5

Bakery (100g or equivalent to a small scone or muffin)

- Crumpet 7.6
- Muffin or scone 8.2
- Pikelet 10
- Lamington 12

Cereal (50g or half a cup)

- Rolled oats 0.9
- All Bran 3.8
- Natural muesli 4.1
- Cornflakes 8.8
- Rice Bubbles 10.9

Dairy (100g/ml)

- Milk 0.3

- Soy milk 0.9
- Yoghurt 1.2
- Mousse 2.4
- Condensed milk 9.7

Fruit (100g or approx. 1 small apple)

- Temperate fruits, e.g. peach, apple, pear and citrus 0.9
- Dried apricots 1.2
- Grapes, kiwifruit
- Mango 3.2
- Raisins 13.2
- Dates 19.1

Legumes (100g approx. half a cup)

- Soybeans 0.3
- Kidney, Mung beans, Lentils 0.9
- Baked beans 1.5

Nuts (35g or a small handful)

- Almond, Brazil, Walnut 0
- Peanut 0.3
- Cashew 0.6

Pasta (180g a medium serving)

- Fettucine (contains egg) 4.7
- Instant noodles 5.3

- Pasta 6.5

Protein and fat-rich foods (any weight)

- Meat, fish, cheese, eggs, seafood 0

Rice (100g)

- Most brown rice 3.5
- High amylose 4.1
- Basmati 4.4
- Calrose brown 6.5
- Sushi rice 7.5
- Jasmine 8.8

Vegetables (100g a small serving)

- Avocado, lettuce, capsicum 0
- Broccoli, cabbage 0.9
- Taro, carrot 1.5
- Peas 3.2
- Sweetcorn 3.5
- Potato 4.1
- Parsnip 4.4

THE EFK WAY

We will now take you through what the key elements are, and some tips and tricks to help you to know *how to make the right food choices anytime, anywhere.*

The Key Elements

Your ultimate goal, wherever possible, is to eat a sustaining mix of protein, fat and carbohydrate for every meal and snack. This keeps you fuller for longer, and with sustained energy and normal blood-sugar levels.

By comparison, if you only eat simple carbohydrate food like a muffin or a scone, you will digest this quickly, have a rush of glucose, high blood-sugar levels and will soon be hungry.

Having your *PFC Table* handy on your phone at all times will help you to learn what all the different combinations are.

The beauty of EFK is that it always comes back to this one big idea of keeping your blood-sugar levels under control.

How to make the right food choices – anytime, anywhere

Engage your senses

- Texture and weight – always look for heavier, firm to hard textured food wherever possible.
- Do a weight test with cereals. Pick up a bag of rolled oats and compare it with a box of cornflakes.
- Do the same with a heavy grain bread versus a white bread loaf. Compare their textures.

- *An exception* – Although Bran cereals are quite light, they have high levels of fibre and digest slowly.

The EFK 'How Much' test

If you are only having small amounts of delicious gravies, sauces, dressings and dips – just enjoy. They have very little effect on the overall result. This is our 'How much' test and is very liberating.

At the Supermarket

- Have your PFC table handy and take time at the supermarket to familiarise yourself with the different combinations in the various sections.
- *It is the overall carbohydrate numbers on the 'Nutrition Information' labels that are important, not just the sugar.* e.g. Cornflakes may show 5/100 grams of sugar, and the carbohydrate will be up to 75/100 grams, and will have many times more impact on your blood-sugar levels than the sugar.
- Fruit and vegetables = complex carbohydrate – firm textured and lots of fibre. Slow digesting and produce few tsp of sugar.
    - Exceptions to this – Bananas have a soft texture, digest quickly and will raise blood-sugar levels. Eat half a banana with some protein and fat-rich food, like a few almond nuts or a piece of cheese. Dried fruit like raisins, dates and sultanas. Starchy vegetables like potatoes, kumara and parsnip

- Fish and seafood, meat and dairy products = protein and fat. Slow digesting and have no effect on blood-sugar levels.
- Use your PFC table to work out how other sections stack up.
- To pick a sustaining bread, cereal, bar or cracker biscuits, check out their weight and textures.

Instructions for pre or Type 2 diabetics on oral medication or insulin injections

- As you make food and drink changes to decrease your overall teaspoons of sugar (tsps) in your diet your blood-sugar levels will decrease.
- This can cause hypos which are potentially dangerous. You should carry barley sugars, jelly babies or similar sweets with you at all times.
- If you feel light headed or dizzy you should immediately have one or more of these sweets and take your blood-sugar levels as soon as possible.

Set targets

- As your blood-sugar levels decrease you can set targets for reducing medication. This should be decided upon before any change of diet with your GP or consultant.
- Normal ranges are: Before meals – 4-7mmol/L, after meals – 5-10mmol/L, Bedtime – 6-10mmol/L.
- If you are at the lower end of these ranges, medication

can be reduced according to guidelines that have been set by your GP.
- Review progress with your GP or consultant regularly. If you are on an automatic delivery system (AID) no action is required.

Note: Your safety is paramount. If you are in doubt about your health at any time please call your health professionals for advice.

This method can be life-changing, enjoy your journey and try to be as consistent as possible to achieve the best results.

FINALLY

I hope you have enjoyed 'The EFK Method' and have gained some clarity on what nutrition is all about and how to make the right food choices. In my experience even two or three changes can make a big difference.

After a bit of practice in your regular food service outlets you will become familiar with how it all works and if you are trying to lose weight or improve a diabetic condition you will soon see improvements.

The key to success is to make any changes to your food and lifestyle a permanent part of your life.

3

BREAKING UP LONG PERIODS OF SITTING

Researchers find that there is a clear link between people who sit for long periods and chronic health conditions. Your metabolism slows, blood sugar rises, muscles stiffen up and can become weaker, and deep-vein thrombosis (blood clots forming in your veins) can result.

If you have been sitting for forty-five minutes or more, get up and get moving. You could do part of your BAFFS routine and be sure to include some high-intensity activity. Any activity that gets your pulse rate up will work.

Going up and down stairs, star jumps, skipping or any other activity like this that you do regularly. Two or three minutes are all you need. This may include three or four 20 to30-second bursts with a short break in between.

A good question is how long you should sit for in total each day. A recent study by The Baker Heart and Diabetes Institute of Melbourne has come up with some useful guidelines.

Recently they put activity trackers on 2400 people from the

Netherlands to discover how long they sat, stood and exercised for each day. They also did a health check on each person. They found that the ideal daily balance for optimal health was about six hours of sitting and a little over five hours for standing.

They also suggested that up to four hours of different types of exercise was optimal. I think that this would be outside the scope of what most people could achieve on a daily basis, particularly with anyone who works a five-day week, unless their work was of a manual or similar type of occupation.

My view is that the most important aspect in striking the right balance is to be always aware of how your day is going with regard to the length of your sitting periods and overall physical activity levels for the day.

If you have a sedentary occupation, it is even more critical to be breaking up your long sitting periods with different forms of exercise, with particular regard to getting yourself puffing two or three times a day.

It is quite useful to have a number to aim for and so I kept a rough track of my overall sitting times for a few days. This was between six and seven hours, which I though was quite good.

You could use that six hours or so as a benchmark and see how you get on. I think a good one would be to sit for no longer than half the hours you are up during the day before you go to bed.

I am up for about fifteen hours on average and so I would aim for no more than seven and a half hours total sitting each day. I would then be happy if I beat that.

Although useful as a guideline, I would not try for anything too exact, more something that you can keep a rough track of and be aware of.

Active sitting

There is a range of active sitting chairs and devices which help you to actually move while you are seated. One of these, for example, is an air-filled rubber balance cushion which you can sit on.

If you are a sedentary worker or spend many hours sitting, one of these would be worth considering.

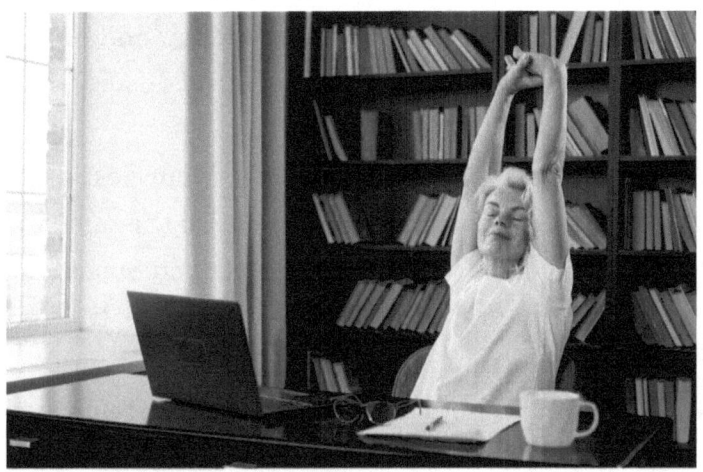

However, you can also remain active by exercising while sitting on an ordinary chair at a desk. I have not been able to find any reference to this simple idea on the internet. All of the focus is on the active chairs.

I shall therefore say that it is a unique and effective concept to keep you exercising without having to leave your desk.

Here are a few ideas examples and you can easily add your own by using a bit of imagination. Exercises will be from both standing and sitting positions.

- Chair stands – Hands on your desk or edge of your seat

and push up to standing position and sit back down and repeat a few times.
- If you pause in the middle of this exercise above, you can hold a squat for a short time.
- You can do the four-stage head and neck stretches we have detailed earlier.
- Twist your trunk to the right and hold and rest your right elbow on the top of the back of your chair and hold for a few seconds. Repeat on the left side and do a few repetitions.
- Place the fingers of both hands under your desk and pull upwards and hold for a few seconds. Do the same by putting your hands on top of the desk and pushing down. Excellent isometric exercises for your biceps, triceps and related muscle groups in your shoulders and core.
- With fists up at shoulder height do rapid air punches with alternate arms.
- Lace your fingers of both hands together and extend these above your head with arms straight. You should feel your whole spine extending.
- Raise your left leg up off the ground and hold for five seconds and repeat with your right leg. Repeat a few times.
- Touch your toes a few times.
- Do a few star jumps.

By doing some of these and adding your own, you are actually exercising and stretching many muscle groups, getting your heart rate up a bit and livening up many of your body's processes.

Spending a couple of minutes doing this every forty-five minutes or so would be very beneficial.

I would like to see this concept developed more fully and it could become a standard in many workplaces. It could eventually be called 'the art of not sitting still'.

4
DRINK FRESH WATER REGULARLY

Dehydration can cause cells to shrink and make it more difficult for your body to regulate temperature. Prolonged dehydration can result in organ failure, and there is also a strong link to a loss of cognitive function.

Astonishingly, our body's composition is approximately 60 per cent water. You need to regularly top up to keep at about this level.

If you struggle to drink water regularly and just have a glass when you remember, it is time to break this habit. You are likely to be damaging your body and risking the early onset of a chronic condition.

It is important to realise that many foods contain a high percentage of water, e.g. some fruits and vegetables are up to 80 per cent.

How much water is enough?

Start to keep track of your urine's colour. If you are well hydrated, it will be pale yellow in colour. If the yellow becomes darker, you will need a top-up.

Obviously, the air temperature and the type of activity that you are involved in are factors in the amount of water you need. A good start to any day is to have a glass of water after you get up and check your urine colour after breakfast. During the day, have a bottle or a glass of water handy wherever you may be and get used to topping up regularly.

You should be able to sense if you are dehydrated as you may feel tired or drowsy and lack energy.

If you do have a problem with drinking water regularly, it will require a concentrated effort over a couple of months using some of the tips above to get the habit. *Staying hydrated is crucial to your ongoing good health.*

5
BUILDING RESILIENCE

You will have already read about building resilience. I have included a short summary below and suggest that you see Chapter 14 – Building Resilience if you require more details.

The definition of resilience is your ability to cope with and bounce back from life's challenges.

If you are a very resilient person, you will still experience all the physical and psychological fears that a less resilient person will feel. You will just be better prepared to deal with them and bounce back more quickly.

To establish a new habit which helps you to build resilience, read through these notes and decide on which areas you can improve. Work out ways of doing this and make the changes. Practise them regularly to establish your new habit.

Considering that our complex lives in today's world can be full of difficulties, your ability to be resilient will play a massive part in your life. And it can mean the difference between having a happy, well-connected and contented life or the absolute opposite.

While resilience may perhaps be an innate genetic quality it also involves the learning of skills.

TEN TRAITS OF RESILIENT PEOPLE

These are not in any particular order of importance.

1. **You are optimistic and positive most of the time** and have a great attitude to life. This sort of attitude is a real asset when things get tough and you are likely to be quite a naturally resilient type.
2. **You will place considerable importance on being physically fit** and are likely to be quite proficient in each of the five BAFFS. This is a real asset when the going gets tough.
3. **You mostly live in the present** and are present in your day-to-day relationships with friends and family.
4. **Resilient people are very likely to be good listeners.** When you are talking to them, they will be giving you their full and undivided attention. As we have just discussed, they are present. *People who are poor listeners miss out on so much.* They are often distracted by other things that are going on in their mind or around them.
5. **You are flexible, know your limits and are able to make other plans.** You may have set your heart on something and worked hard to achieve it. It will not always come to pass; sometimes you miss out. Resilience gives you the ability to accept this, maybe learn some lessons from it, and move on.

6. **You like spending time on your own.** This sounds counter-intuitive to the other resilience measure of being well connected. *What it means is that in our busy, complex and connected-up lives, time on our own can be a wonderful change.* On the other hand, a person who craves others' attention and company at all times may have some self-worth issues.
7. **You have the ability to say no.** It can be so difficult when someone close to you puts you on the spot and you just do not like to say no, even though you know that you probably should. When you are put on the spot, say you will come back to them. This buys you time to make a more considered decision.
8. **You have purpose in your life.** Having a reason for being, and a clear purpose in life, is an absolute cornerstone for being a resilient person.
9. **You are grateful for what you have**. Focus on all the positive aspects of your life.
10. **You are well connected to your friends and family and value the day-to-day contact you have with them.**

Thanks for taking on The Don't Act Your Age Challenge.

If you are ready to make a few permanent changes to form new lifestyle habits, you will be very likely to succeed.

Success in this case can be life-changing and offer you many more years of good health. You're worth it!

WHAT TO DO NOW?

You should now have your written list of areas that you want to focus on and the various actions, stretches and exercises that you have selected.

Atomic Habits – Write down a list of your current daily habits and attach some of your selected actions, stretches and exercises to some of these.

If you are unsure of how to proceed, I have compiled below an example of the framework of one person's notes that you could use to write down your own selections. This could be helpful if you want to have a clear picture of how you were going to tackle your challenge.

Sam Jones

BAFFS
Balance – standing on one leg (includes putting on socks and trousers), heel to toe, walking along lines.
Flexibility – Head and neck four-way stretch, Child's Pose, Downward Dog, touching toes and windscreen wipers.
Strength – Press-ups, planking, squats and biceps and triceps curls.
Fitness – Always take the stairs, add hills to my walks, and skip with a rope for two minutes.
Nutrition – The EFK Method
Change from cornflakes to rolled oats, change to wholegrain bread, cut down on rice and potatoes and sushi portions.
Hydration
Keep an eye on urine colour, drink a glass of water before I get up, and have a bottle on my desk.
Active sitting
Do this routine every forty minutes while at desk – ten chair stands, fifty air punches, head and neck stretch x 2, touch toes x 3, ten star jumps.
Resilience
Talk to at least one friend or family member each day and be more positive.
Atomic Habits
Everyday habits Atomic habits
Wake up Drink glass of water

Get dressed Stand on one leg to put trousers and socks on

Breakfast Head and neck stretch while microwaving oats

Brush teeth Stand on one leg

Walk to work Add in a hill, walk on lines, do heel-to-toe balance

Morning work Do strength exercises to break up sitting periods

Lunch Phone friend and family member

Afternoon work As in morning, do active sitting routine every forty minutes

Dinner Cut down on spuds and rice

TV Do remaining stretches and two-minute skip with rope

Note: You can use this same format to set up your own routine.

Thanks for taking up the challenge, we hope that you will enjoy the journey, become biologically younger and add more healthy years to your life.

IN CONCLUSION

It has been both a privilege and a challenge to write this book and I have met some amazing people along the way. I hope you have enjoyed it and will also gain some life benefits.

I will leave you with two final insights. The first is a remarkable and scary statistic which highlights how the power of your mind can determine your future health and happiness.

A recent Oregon University study found that people who took a really positive attitude towards ageing were likely to live on average seven and a half years longer than their more pessimistic counterparts.

And the second, *you brush your teeth every day, don't you?* Remember that there are all of the other parts of your body just crying out for the same regular care.

Your incredible body and mind never stop ticking over, keeping you moving, breathing, thinking, digesting food, excreting waste, and so much more.

Regularity is vital – Doing two gym or yoga sessions a week is all very well. Your body still has to keep going for those other five days. Paying attention to your BAFFS and other key routines daily or as often as possible will really pay off.

If you keep following the basic principles of my approach, you will achieve some new lifestyle habits. And your body will love you for it.

Finally, if you deliberately 'don't act your age' and try to live younger, you are very likely to succeed!

ABOUT THE AUTHOR

Leigh is a fit eighty-two-year-old and a former all-round sportsman, physical education teacher, life coach, rest-home owner, columnist and author of two popular health books.

He is on a mission to both walk-the-talk and talk-the-talk with as many people as possible about their long-term health and fitness.

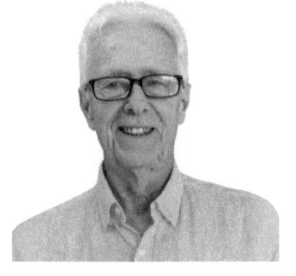

This new book, *Don't Act Your Age*, is the culmination of all these years of wide-ranging experience. It is a natural progression on from his work as founder of the Eat For Keeps programme which has already positively changed the lives of thousands of people with weight and diabetes issues.

https://leighelder.substack.com
leighelderwriter@gmail.com

ABOUT THE AUTHOR

ACKNOWLEDGMENTS

My dear wife Kate who must have thought, here we go again.

Arch Jelley, Margaret Borland, June Weston, Vic Murray, Pat Ryder and Sherilyn Hurman for their generosity in providing their life stories. These have provided many fascinating insights for our readers.

My publisher Martin Taylor who expertly guided me through the publishing process and produced a fine-looking book.

Ryman Healthcare management and staff for being very supportive and providing excellent facilities for my presentations, workshops and the book launch.

Maryvonne Gray for her great support and expert help with a Powerpoint and various media opportunities.

So many health professionals, friends and family encouraging me to get out there again and give this a good crack.

Brian O'Flaherty for such an insightful proofread.

Bob Stevens' generosity in providing me with such a great editing process.

www.ingramcontent.com/pod-product-compliance
Lightning Source LLC
Chambersburg PA
CBHW031237290426
44109CB00012B/332